A COMPARATIVE STUDY ON SELECTED PSYCHO-PHYSICAL FITNESS COMPONENTS OF KABADDI AND KHO-KHO PLAYERS

D1641938

BY
SUNIL KUMAR

Copyright©2022

Book Name: *A Comparative Study on Selected Psycho-Physical Fitness Components of Kabaddi and Kho Kho Players*

TABLE OF CONTENTS

LIST OF TABLES

LIST OF FIGURES

CHAPTER - I

INTRODUCTION

Sport serves vital and important role in social and cultural functioning for each individual. In the last few decades sports have gained tremendous popularity all over the globe. The popularity of sports is still increasing at a fast pace and this happy trend is likely to continue in the future also. The contribution of sports towards the overall welfare of the human society may be capsule in the following points:

a)   Sports help in the all-around development of human personality.

b)   Provide ample and healthy means for recreation and relaxation of human mind and body.

c)   Are effective for rehabilitation and social adjustment to the injured, sick and handicapped.

d)   Provide opportunities for social interaction thereby fostering peace and understanding among different people, nations, races, religion etc.

e)   Perform preventive and curative functions for several diseases and ailments inflicting human body and mind.

f)   Provide healthy and socially acceptable opportunities for the people and nations to complete against each other thereby touching heights to excellence of human endeavor and attainment.

Barrow and Gee (1999) acknowledged that the physical fitness is a complex phenomenon consisting of various factors such as speed, strength, flexibility agility, cardiovascular endurance etc.

Jenson and Fisher (1999) clarified as physical traits are considered as important parameters for athletes (Sprinter) such strength, power, speed, agility, co-ordination, muscular endurance, reaction time, cardiovascular respiratory endurance and flexibility. Since speed, agility, power, co-ordination and reaction time are specific motor traits. These traits are best developed by the repeated practice of the different trainings for which they are needed. The strength, speed, agility co-ordination, power, flexibility contribute to these motor traits.

Strength is a helping element to several performance traits as it contributes to power (Power = Force x Velocity). The increased strength results in the ability to apply more force and thereby it contributes to power; strength is also a factor in muscular endurance, which is the ability of the muscles to resist fatigue whole doing work.

force is required to accelerate the body and its parts rapidly. Also, strength is a factor in running speed because force is required to accelerate the body and keep it in motion at top speed. There is no doubt that lack of sufficient strength is a serious handicap too many would be good players.

Among the most universal and most engrossing of all human pursuits is the attempt to understand the human being. Philosophers, political scientists, sociologists, anthropologists, biologists, physiologists, psychologists- all study man and cast into print the results of their observations. The butcher, baker, and the candlestick maker- all study man, albeit in a casual way, and use the results of their study as a basis for conducting their daily lives. Each of us, in his own way, has studies human beings. And each of us has developed his own view of man.

Psychology deals with all phases of the psychological process, which may be viewed against some perspectives and may consider the general nature of the scientific approach to the study of psychological phenomena. The several studies indicated the following out-comes of their studies:

1. The organism grows and develops over time; the nature and sequences of development help determine the nature and sequences of behavior seen in the psychological process.

2. The human infant has a biological history, a biological and psychological future.

3. On the historical side, the human infant has an evolutionary heredity, a species heredity, and an individual heredity- all represented in the pattern of his genes and chromosomes.

4. His heredity gives the human individual not only a similarity to other organisms but also uniqueness.

5. More than other kind of organism, the human neonate is relatively dependent and his behavior relatively free of instinctual determination.

6. The individual inherits physical traits, capacities, and susceptibilities; and his inherited charactertics have both direct and indirect effects on his behavior.

7. There is evidence that an organism's genetic background may contribute to its capacity to learn; and the human capacity to behave intelligently has a hereditary component.

8. The possibility exists that in some families there may be an inherited susceptibility to schizophrenia.

9. Hereditary and environmental factors interact in many ways to produce the patterns of adjustment we observe.

10. Emotional experiences on the part of mother rats during pregnancy produce emotionally in the offspring.

11. The development of the organism follows a cephalocaudal sequence, a proximaldistal sequence, and sequences of differentiation and integration.

12. There are normal sequence with respect to motor development, language development, and emotional development. All individuals, at least in Western cultures, follow similar sequences; but each develops at his own rate.

13. The functioning of the ductless glands- especially the pituitary, the thyroid, the adrenals, and the gonads- influences significantly the growth of the individual.

14. Learning of certain tasks and skills cannot occur until maturation has redirected the organism; the stage of maturation determines what the organism can learn.

15. Early sensory and perceptual experience, or the lack of it, has a bearing on mature sensory and perceptual abilities.

16. Early physical experiences, such as handling or isolation or stress, have definite effects on the later behavior of animals.

17. There is evidence, though somewhat controversial, that infants deprived of early love and attention show severe personality disturbances.

18. The timing and nature of early child-parent relationship can affect development; at certain critical periods young animals tend to become imprinted on large moving objects, tending to follows these objects about as if there were mothers.

19. Research on the effect of artificial experimental mothers suggests importance of the feel of the mother in the developing attachment to her; infant monkeys with "wire mothers" behave quite differently from these with 'cloth mothers."

Now a day, there has been an ever increasing focus on attention on the study of individual differences in research. In this regard a large number of researchers are engaged in comparing the motor performance of different sections of population in terms of race or otherwise various regional backgrounds. The net results of their finding have been contradictory and there is no unanimity among the research scholars regarding inter-relationship between or the degree of influence.

So far, the selection of potential outstanding sportsmen for social sports has mainly been done in most states/countries by intention or in other words left to the good eye of the concerned physical education teacher or coach. We know from the facts that the ultimate performance of the mature athlete is determined by a large number of factors, such as genetic, nutritional status, climate, sociological and psychological, as well as type of cultural activity and training to which the individual is exposed (Yiglety, 2001).

To develop the motor components of the athletes, training is an essential aspect. The present study was considered with selected training programme so as to compile the physiological characteristics of Kho-Kho players selected from various schools of Delhi. The following trainings were adopted for improvement of motor abilities:

a)   Circuit training

b)   Fartlek training

c)   Sprint and strides

d)   Shuttle Run

e)   Jig-jag Running

force is required to accelerate the body and its parts rapidly. Also, strength is a factor in running speed because force is required to accelerate the body and keep it in motion at top speed. There is no doubt that lack of sufficient strength is a serious handicap too many would be good players.

Among the most universal and most engrossing of all human pursuits is the attempt to understand the human being. Philosophers, political scientists, sociologists, anthropologists, biologists, physiologists, psychologists- all study man and cast into print the results of their observations. The butcher, baker, and the candlestick maker- all study man, albeit in a casual way, and use the results of their study as a basis for conducting their daily lives. Each of us, in his own way, has studies human beings. And each of us has developed his own view of man.

Psychology deals with all phases of the psychological process, which may be viewed against some perspectives and may consider the general nature of the scientific approach to the study of psychological phenomena. The several studies indicated the following out-comes of their studies:

20. The organism grows and develops over time; the nature and sequences of development help determine the nature and sequences of behavior seen in the psychological process.

21. The human infant has a biological history, a biological and psychological future.

22. On the historical side, the human infant has an evolutionary heredity, a species heredity, and an individual heredity- all represented in the pattern of his genes and chromosomes.

23. His heredity gives the human individual not only a similarity to other organisms but also uniqueness.

24. More than other kind of organism, the human neonate is relatively dependent and his behavior relatively free of instinctual determination.

25. The individual inherits physical traits, capacities, and susceptibilities; and his inherited charactertics have both direct and indirect effects on his behavior.

26. There is evidence that an organism's genetic background may contribute to its capacity to learn; and the human capacity to behave intelligently has a hereditary component.

27. The possibility exists that in some families there may be an inherited susceptibility to schizophrenia.

28. Hereditary and environmental factors interact in many ways to produce the patterns of adjustment we observe.

29. Emotional experiences on the part of mother rats during pregnancy produce emotionally in the offspring.

30. The development of the organism follows a cephalocaudal sequence, a proximaldistal sequence, and sequences of differentiation and integration.

31. There are normal sequence with respect to motor development, language development, and emotional development. All individuals, at least in Western cultures, follow similar sequences; but each develops at his own rate.

32. The functioning of the ductless glands- especially the pituitary, the thyroid, the adrenals, and the gonads- influences significantly the growth of the individual.

33. Learning of certain tasks and skills cannot occur until maturation has redirected the organism; the stage of maturation determines what the organism can learn.

34. Early sensory and perceptual experience, or the lack of it, has a bearing on mature sensory and perceptual abilities.

35. Early physical experiences, such as handling or isolation or stress, have definite effects on the later behavior of animals.

36. There is evidence, though somewhat controversial, that infants deprived of early love and attention show severe personality disturbances.

37. The timing and nature of early child-parent relationship can affect development; at certain critical periods young animals tend to become imprinted on large moving objects, tending to follows these objects about as if there were mothers.

38. Research on the effect of artificial experimental mothers suggests importance of the feel of the mother in the developing attachment to her; infant monkeys with "wire mothers" behave quite differently from these with 'cloth mothers."

So far, the selection of potential outstanding sportsmen for social sports has mainly been done in most states/countries by intention or in other words left to the good eye of the concerned physical education teacher or coach. Yiglety (2001) We know from the facts that the ultimate performance of the mature athlete is determined by a large number of factors, such as genetic, nutritional status, climate, sociological and psychological, as well as type of cultural activity and training to which the individual is exposed

To develop the motor components of the athletes, training is an essential aspect. The present study was considered with selected training programme so as to compile the physiological characteristics of Kho-Kho players selected from various schools of Delhi. The following trainings were adopted for improvement of motor abilities:

(a) Circuit training

(b) Fartlek training

(c) Sprint and strides

(d) Shuttle Run

(e) Jig-jag Running

Physical fitness is an attribute required for service in virtually all military forces. Physical fitness comprises two related concepts: general fitness (a state of health and well-being) and specific fitness (a task-oriented definition based on the ability to perform specific aspects of sports or occupations). Physical fitness is generally achieved through exercise, correct nutrition and enough rest. It is an important part of life. In previous years, fitness was commonly defined as the capacity to carry out the day's activities without undue fatigue. However, as automation increased leisure time, changes in lifestyles following the industrial revolution rendered this definition insufficient.

These days, physical fitness is considered a measure of the body's ability to function efficiently and effectively in work and leisure activities, to be healthy, to resist hypo-kinetic diseases, and to meet emergency situations. Physical fitness' is the capacity to do prolong hard work and recover to the same state of health in short duration of time. This is the result of the degree of strength, speed endurance, agility, power and flexibility one possesses. These elements of physical fitness are useful for different games and sports. Physical fitness depends on several factors such as heredity, hygienic living, nutrition and body maneuvers of an individual. Amongst these, body man overs ever play an important role.

Different games provided to do the body activities, differently. Kabaddi and Kho- Kho players are equally conductive to developing these skills amongst players. The theory of coordinative abilities is though it is rapidly getting recognition in the world of sports. However, there is no general agreement regarding the number of coordinative abilities required for sports.

Components of Physical Fitness:

The President's Council on Physical Fitness and Sports—a study group sponsored by the government of the United States—declines to offer a simple definition of physical fitness. Instead, it developed the following chart:(http://en.wikipedia.org/wiki/Motor_coordination)

Physiological Components	Health Related Components	Skill Related Components	Sports Related Components
• Metabolic	• Body Composition	• Agility	• Team Sport
• Morphological	• Cardiovascular Fitness	• Balance	• Individual Sport
• Bone Integrity	• Flexibility	• Coordination	• Life-time
• Other	• Muscular Endurance	• Power	• Other
	• Muscle Strength	• Speed	
		• Reaction Time	
		• Other	

Accordingly, a general purpose of the physical fitness programme must address to the following essential and core nature of components:

- Cardiovascular Endurance
- Flexibility Score
- Strength
- Muscular Endurance (Stamina)
- Body Composition
- General Skill Ability

However, along with these essential components, a comprehensive fitness program that is tailored to an individual will probably focus on one or more specific skills, and on age or health-related needs such as bone health. Many sources also cite mental, social and emotional health as an important part of overall fitness. This is often presented in textbooks as a triangle made up of three points, which represent physical, emotional, and mental fitness. Physical fitness can also prevent or treat many chronic health conditions brought on by unhealthy lifestyle or aging. Working out can also help people sleep better. To stay healthy it's important to participate in physical activity.

Specific fitness- Specific or task-oriented fitness is a person's ability to perform in a specific activity with a reasonable efficiency as a sports, or military services. A specific training prepares athletes to perform well in their sports competition. The following are few of the examples to understand the concept:

- 400 m sprint: in a sprint the athlete must be trained to work an aerobically through-out the race.
- Marathon: in this case the athlete must be trained to work aerobically and their endurance must be built-up to a maximum.

- Many fire fighters and police officers undergo regular fitness testing to determine if they are capable of the physically demanding tasks required of the job.

Members of the United States Army and Army National Guard must be able to pass the Army Physical Fitness Test (APFT).

Since, every sport has different type of energy requirement depending on the nature and duration of the activity, so it is vitally important to develop the reservoir of energy sources accordingly. Kumari (2007) It has been established beyond doubt, "Much of the human physiology is controlled by human physical fitness and that physiological preparation in sport is consequential in the absence of study human performance as it is related to competitive sport. Physical fitness is the result of regular physical activity, proper diet and nutrition, and proper rest for physical within the parameters allowed by the genome.

It usually happens frequently that teams, as well as individual player, don't produce the performance in a much which would normally be expected of them, despite their excellent physical conditions. Experience has also frequently shown that team or players, that are considered rather weak, may play above themselves & are capable of producing outstanding performance. The reasons for this lie in the realm of Psychology. The good Coach knows that the team's or the player's ability does not depend merely on physical, technical & tactical qualities, but also on

Psychological consideration influencing these, so as to benefit performance, is one of the many important tasks that the coach has to master. Narang (2003).

The physiology is a branch of biology concerned with the function of the body. (Thibodeav et. al. 1993) Physiology is the science that treats the functions of the living organism and its parts. The term "Physiology" is a combination of two Greek words Physics means "Nature" and Logos means "Science of Study". Simply stated, it is the study of physiology that helps to understand how the body works.

Moran (1996) Sports psychology, the youngest of the sport science, is concerned with the psychological effect derived from participation. Today many outlets & Coaches look to sport psychology for a competitive edge by seeking psychological training Programme in order to learn among other thing, way to manage, competitive stress, central concentration, improve confidence & increase communication skill & team harmony. Competitive sports provides psychologist with many fascinating opportunities to explore the success with which people can control their own mental processes in the face of adversity. If paying attention is viewed as an effort to exert control over what we perceive & do, then the study of concentration in athletes offers a potentially fruitful new avenue for the study of how the mind works.

Statement of the Problem

The present study was of the comparative nature of research work. The statement of problem was formally sated as: **A COMPARATIVE STUDY ON SELECTED PSYCHO-PHYSICAL FITNESS COMPONENTS OF KABADDI AND KHO-KHO PLAYERS OF DELHI SCHOOLS.**

Objectives of the Study:

The main objective of the present study is to find-out the difference between Kabaddi and Kho-Kho players at senior secondary school level in regards to their psycho-physical variables. The main purpose is more elaborately defended as the flowing sub-objectives:

- To find-out the different between physical fitness components of Kabaddi and Kho-Kho players such as speed, explosive strength, cardiovascular endurance, coordinative ability, and flexibility.
- To find-out the difference between the Kabaddi and Kho-Kho in sports competition anxiety, concentration level and psychomotor ability.

Hypotheses of the Study:

After going through the review of the related literature, the investigator was of the opinion to apply null hypothesis for the present investigation. This was done due to very less review found in this area and moreover, the related literature was not able to decide any directional hypothesis. The null hypothesis set and stated as below:

1. There will be no significant difference in physical fitness factors of Kabaddi players and Kho-Kho players.
2. There will be no significant difference in psychological factors of Kabaddi and Kho-Kho players.

Delimitations of the Study:

The present study was the following delimitations:

- The study was delimited to purposively select 100 male subjects age ranging from 16 to 19 years of Delhi schools, who has participated in Inter-Zonal and School National (SGFI) Junior National of Kabaddi and Kho-Kho competition.

- The study was further delimited out of 100 male players' at schools levels a total of 50 male players of Kabaddi and 50 male Kho-Kho players were selected.

- The investigation was delimited to selected variables such as physical and psychological parameters as under:-

1. Anthropometric Components:

    a. Height

    b. Body weight

    c. Body Mass Index (BMI)

2. Physical Fitness Components:

    a. **Speed:** 40 m. Sprint

    b. **Explosive Strength:** Standing Broad Jump

    c. **Cardiovascular Endurance:** 12 min. Run/Walk Test

    d. **Coordinative Ability:** 4X10 m. Shuttle Run

    e. **Flexibility:** Sit and Reach Test

3. Psychological Components:

The Psychological abilities measure with selected tests as under-

    a. **Psycho-motor Ability:** Eye-hand Coordination Test

    b. **Concentration:** Grid Concentration Test

    c. **Sports Competition Anxiety Test** (SCAT)

Limitations of the Study:

The research scholar has anticipated few limitations for the present study. The findings of the study may be understood by considering the following limitations during the study faced by the scholar:

1. Availability of small number of sample size was one of the limitations of the study.
2. Sophisticated testing equipment for exercises was also one of the limitations for the present study.
3. Individual differences among the subjects and other factors such as- Life Style, dietary habits, daily routine, were also considered limitations for the present study.
4. Social stigma /religion, culture and social practices of the subjects in study may also be considered as Limitation for the Study.

Definitions and Explanations of the Terms Used:

Physical Fitness:

Clarke defined, 'Physical Fitness' as 'the ability of carry-out daily task with vigor and alertness without undue fatigue and with ample energy to enjoy leisure time pursuits to meet unforeseen emergencies'. The American Association for Health, Physical Education, and Recreation defines total fitness as: .... that state which characterizes the degree to which the person is able to function.

Psychological Fitness- It refers to controlling the mental factors or abilities to optimal use of psychological aspects/factors of sports performance in sports competition.

Concentration- It is the ability to concentrate or focused on an object or assigned work for the required length of duration.

Sports Competition Anxiety: The sports competition anxiety considers as the interaction between the personality/individual differences in tendency to become anxious along with varied situational factor in competitive sports.

Coordinative Ability: Coordinative ability is the ability of the body to maintain the balance of the body of coordinated movements of the different body parts. To judge the differentiation ability and to perform a particular movement with less efforts and least expenditure of the energy of the body, stores in muscles and liver.

Coordinative ability is understood as relatively stabilized and generalized patterns of motor control and regulation process. These enable the sportsman to do a group of movements with better quality and effect".

Speed: It is the ability to cover the assigned distance in minimum possible time. It is the performance pre-requisite to do motor actions under given conditions (movement task, external factors, individual pre-requisite) in minimum of time.

It defines the capacity of moving a limb or part of the body's lever system or the whole body with greatest possible velocity without or with loading- i.e. velocity of discuss arm with or without discuss. But improvement in speed of arm may not improve performance till achieve synchronized movement.

Strength- It is the ability to act against the resistance. "Strength is the ability to overcome resistance or to act against the resistance" or "Strength, or the ability to express force, is a basic physical characteristic that determine performanceefficiency in sport".

Endurance: It defined asit is ability to perform in presence of fatigue or tiredness or "Ability to resist fatigue". Harre (1986) defined it, "As to the resistance ability to fatigue". Thiess & Schnabel (1987) "Ability to do sports movements with the desired quality and speed under conditions of fatigue".

Flexibility- It is a range or amplitude of the moment at a specific joint of body parts. It is related with quality of muscles, tendons and ligaments at particular joint.

Significance of the Study:

The findings of the study may have the following significance and contribution to the related field. The findings of the study have the significance of self-assessment of physical fitness abilities factors and psychological aspects of Kabaddi and Kho-Kho players:

1. The study seeks to bring-out the significance through the comparison of these factors between the of Kabaddi and Kho-Kho players.
2. The study has the significance of making of training schedule for the players, coaches, trainers and physical education teachers for Kabaddi and Kho-Kho players to develop psycho-physical fitness of sportsman.
3. The study contrary to above has the significance to select the of Kabaddi and Kho-Kho players on the basis of the evolution of psycho-physical fitness abilities factors as proceeded by the individuals.
4. The present study has also the significance of proposing guideline and index for future researchers in the field of Kabaddi and Kho-Kho.

CHAPTER - II

REVIEW OF RELATED LITERATURE

The research scholar made an attempt to present a summary review of the related literature, which may be helpful in understanding the basic trends available and to bring-out the meaningful outcomes of the present study. The scholar tried his level best to gather the best available literature. For this purpose, he has visited number of libraries like: Indira Gandhi Institute of Physical Education and Sports Sciences (University of Delhi), Central Institute of Education (University of Delhi), Central Library (University of Delhi), Lakshmibai National University of Physical Education (Deemed University, Gwalior, M. P.). In addition to the above sources, the investigator searched various related websites on internet and available personal and supervisor's literature etc.

This chapter includes reviews of related literature for the present study which has been taken by the researcher. The scholar has undertaken the extensive searchfor the reviews and has collected the following reviews of the critical literature:

Siddhu and Kumari (1993) suggested about the relationship between activity and blood pressure level among 500 adult individual of Punjab positive association between physical activity and Systolic and Diastolic blood pressure were observed in the study further in majority of age groups person with light physical activity show marked higher incidence of hypertension than their medium and heavy physical activity counterpart.

Bhomik (1997) conducted a comparative study on selected physiological parameter between Soccer and Kabaddi players. The purpose of the study was to compare and contrast the selected physiological parameters between soccer and Kabaddi players. Total 30 players from the Kabaddi and soccer (15 from each) were selected randomly land only from the Intercollegiate terms of Amravati University. The physiological parameters selected as criterion were blood pressure, vital capacity and resting pulse rate. The "t" test was computed to find out the significance differences between the mean. It was concluded that Kabaddi players were significantly superior in vital capacity whereas soccer players were significantly superior in resting pulse rate in comparison to their counterpart but in case of blood pressure non- significance difference were found between the two groups.

Jones and et al. (2001) conducted a study with a purpose to extend existing sport psychological research by developing a more comprehensive athlete attitudinal survey the sport performance inventory (SPI). A multiple item survey consisting of sport related attitudinal items was distributed to 274 students athletes enrolled in a large division Midwestern university. A Principal components analysis with varimax rotation performance on the original survey items resulted in an 83 item survey items resulted in an 83 items survey with 6 interpretable factors: competitiveness, team orientation, mental toughness emotional control, positive attitude, and safety consciousness, all subscales demonstrated adequate items discriminate ability internal consistency important statistically significant differences between college invoice and male / female athletes were found : (1) college athletes were found to have a higher SPI composite than novice athletes : (2) college athletes were found to have a more positive attitude than novice athletes; (3) college athletes were more competitive than novice athletes; (4) female were more

21

them oriented than males; & (5) novice males were more competitive than novice female, while female were more competitive than college males.

Loehrs (1996) constructed Psychological Performance Inventory (PPI), the most influential mental toughness instrument measured through the seven most important psychological factors that reflect mental toughness: self-confidence, negative energy, attention control, visual and imagery control, motivation, positive energy and attitude control. The PPI is a 42 item self- report instrument designed to measure factors that reflect mental toughness. All questions in the PPI were answered using a 6-point Likhert type scale, ranging from '1' (False) to '6' (True).

Davis et al. (1998) investigated mental toughness and assessed casual explanations for positive and negative reactions to imagined events using an attributional style questionnaire pessimistic explanatory style on this scale were a risk factor for negative affect and behavior following negative events. 38 elite athletes (minimum age 17.8 years) in Ice-hockey were rated for mental toughness shows. Composite explanations of negative events that was more internal, stable and global for players above the median. The results suggest that a pessimistic explanatory style may benefit hockey performance.

Middleton et al. (2004) constructed the Mental Toughness Inventory (MTI). The MTI is a 67-item instrument designed to measure twelve components of mental toughness along with global mental toughness (i.e., 13 factors in total). The factors measured include self-efficacy, Future Potential, Mental Self-Concept, Task Familiarity, Value, Personal Best Motivation, Goal commitment, Task specific attention, and perseverance, Positivity, Positive Comparisons, Stress minimization and Global Mental Toughness.

22

Gharote (1992) studied the effect of Yogic exercises on the strength and endurance of the abdominal muscles of the females after giving three weeks yogic exercises. The result was that he found significant increase in the strength and endurance of the abdominal muscle of the females.

Dhanaraj, Aubert (1994) studied the effect of yoga and the 5 BX fitness plan on selected physiological parameters. The results indicated increases in basal metabolic rate, tidal volume in basal state, T-4 Thyroxin, hemoglobin, hematocrit, and RBC count PWC 130, Vital capacity, and chest expansion, breath holding time and flexibility after yogic training.

Barrett and Fisher (1997) determined the relationship between selected variable of physical fitness and academic achievement for elementary and secondary students specially each variable of physical fitness, which included a mile run, skinfold fat measurement of the triceps and subscapular site, sit ups and a sit and reach activity was corrected with standardized method and reading scores. The instrument which was used is AAHPERD. Health related physical fitness test. The result was that there was significant for any grade levels, based upon the findings.

Birkel and Edgren (2000) conducted a study with a purpose to find-out the vital capacity of the lungs which is a critical component of good health. Vital capacity is an important concern for those with asthma, heart conditions, and lung ailments; those who smoke; and those who have no known lung problems. Objective: To determine the effects of Yoga postures and breathing exercise on vital capacity.Design of the study,using the Spiro-meter, researchers measured vital capacity. Vital capacity determinants were taken near the beginning and end of two

17 week semesters. No control group was used. Setting: Midwestern University Yoga classes taken for college credit participants.

A total of 287 college students, 89 men and 198 women, Intervention: subjects were taught Yoga poses, breathing techniques, and relaxation in two 50 minutes class meetings for 15 weeks. Main Out-come Measures were: Vital capacity over time for smoker's asthmatics, and those with no known lung disease. Results: The study showed a statistically significant (P< .001) improvement in vital capacity across all categories over time. Conclusions: It is not known whether these findings were the result or Yoga poses, breathing techniques, relation, or other aspects of exercise in the subject's life. The subject's adherence to attending class was 99.96%. The large number of 287 subjects is considered to be a valid number for a study of this type. These findings are consistent withother research studies reporting the positive effect of Yoga on the vital capacity of the lungs.

Stancak et al. (1991) studied on cardio-vascular and respiratory changes during yogic breathing exercise kapalabhati (KB) in 7 advanced yoga practitioners.The exercise consisted in fast shallow abdominal respiration movements at about 2 Hz frequencies. Blood pressure, ECG and respiration were recorded continuously during three 5 min periods of KB and during Pre and post – KB resting periods. The beat-to-beat series of systolic blood pressure (SBP) and diastolic blood pressure (DBP). R-R intervals and respiration were analyzed by spectral analysis of time series.

The mean absolute power was calculated three frequency bands of spontaneous respiration, band of 0.1 Hz rhythm and the low-frequency band greater than 15 S in all spectra. The mean modulus calculated between SBP and R-R intervals was used as a parameter of baro receptor- cardiac reflex sensitivity (BRS). Heart rate increased by a beat per minute during KB,SBP, and DBP increased during KB by 15 and 6 mm Hg respectively.

All frequency bands of R-R interval variability were reduced in KB. Also the BRS parameter was reduced in KB. The amplitude of the high frequency oscillations in SBP and DBP increased during KB. The low frequency blood pressure oscillations were increased after KB. The results point to decreased cardiac vagal tone during KB which was due to change in respiratory pattern and due to decreased sensitivity of arterial spirometer. Decreased respiratory rate and increased SBP and low frequency blood pressure. Oscillations after KB suggest a differentiated pattern of vegetatine activation and inhabitation associated with KB exercise.

Reilly et. al. (1984) conducted a study on ten subjects to investigate the circadian rhythm in heart rate at rest, immediately pre-exercise, during sub-maximal and maximal exercise on a cycle ergo meter and during recovery post exercise under control conditions at 03:00, 15:00 and 21:00 hours. The study showed a significant circadian rhythm for resting heart rate lying supine and sitting pre-exercise (p<0.05) peak values being measured at 15:00 hours. The acro-phase in the oral temperature, rhythm at 17:39 hours was not significantly out of phase with that of resting during sub-maximal exercise (150 w) and at the maximal rate (p<0.05) the amplitude of rhythm was attended at maximum.

Rating of perceived exertion at sub-maximal and maximal exercise intensities and time to exhaustion or ergo meter test doesn't vary significantly with time of the day (P<0.05), The result revealed a significant rhythm for recovery heart rate in minutes 2, 3, 4, and 5 post-exercise (p<0.05) Thus the study suggests that the cireadian rhythm in heart rates responses to exercise to be considered when a heart rate variable is to be used as an index of physiological strain.

Atkinson et.al. (1993) compared circadian rhythm in physiological, subjective; and performance measures between groups exhibiting different levels of habitual activity: fourteen male subjects; aged 19-29 years were assigned to a physically active (group-I, n=7) or a physical inactive (group-II; n=7) group on the basis of leisure time physical inactive: Rectal temperature, oral temperature; resting pulse rate, subjective arousal and sleepiness were measured a 2:00, 6:00, 10:00, 14:00 18:00 and 20:00 hours in a counter balanced sequence for each subject whole body flexibility; back and leg strength grip strength, flight time in a vertical jump, physical working capacity teat (pwc150) and self- chosen work rate were recorded at each time point.

The data were subjected to the group casino method. The results confirm with physical performance measures that rhythm amplitudes are higher for physically fit subjects. This could be attributed to greater early-morning through in the measures for active individuals. Since the subjects were sedentary immediately prior to testing, it is possible that these finding are training effect of physical activity.

Roy (1994) has conducted a study on the body size, strength, muscular endurance and power of top flight team in England Rugby and Soccer players. Mean superiority's by team were amateur Rugby players in muscular endurance and the professional Rugby Players in weight and vertical jump, amateur soccer players in push-ups and pull ups and muscular endurance, professional soccer players in back strength and sit ups. The offensive amateur and professional Rugby players were superior to the defensive soccer players were superior to the forwards in body weight and height and the amateur defensive players were superior in strength index.

Debnath (1990) concluded his study with the purpose to generalize, compare and contrast some selected physiological variables and body composition among Football, Kho-Kho and Table-tennis players. Total 45 inter-collegiate players (15 from each game) of Amravati University were selected randomly. Selected physiological and body composition were measured and analysed by f- ratio test. It was concluded that Football players had significantly higher hemoglobin content, resting pulse rate and vital capacity and balance body composition in comparison to Kho- Kho and Table -tennis players.

Ramaden (1995) investigates to examine the maximal oxygen consumption (Vo2 max), maximal anaerobic power, body composition and the state trait anxiety, characteristics of Kuwaiti world cup soccer players. The Kuwaiti teams exhibited moderately high aerobic (51.9 ml/kg min) and anaerobic (119.6 kg/m/sec.) power both value being significantly higher than college norms. The world cup soccer players revealed a significantly higher value in anger factors.

Ray (1990) conducted a study on the status of physical fitness and physiological parameter of offensive and defensive players of soccer and hockey. Who is purpose of the study is to find-out the status of selected physical fitness and physiological parameters of offensive and defensive players of Football and Hockey. Sixty inter-collegiate male offensive and defensive players of Football and Hockey were selected randomly from the Degree College of Physical Education, Amravati. Six selected physical and physiological parameters were measured and recorded.The 'F' ratio was computed to find-out the significance differences. It was concluded that there were significance differenced in vertical jump 50 Yard Dash and pulse rate whereas, non-significant differences were observed in vital capacity, 12 min. run/walk, and blood pressure of Football and Hockey players.

Mohammad et al. (1991) conducted a study on selective physiological, psychological and Anthropometric characteristics of Kuwaiti world cup soccer team. The purpose of this study was to examine the maximal oxygen consumption Vol. 2 max) body composition some type characteristic of Kuwaiti world cup soccer team. The (Vol. 2 max) was determined using a progressive cycle-ergo meter; the skin fold was estimated by skim folds and somatotype was by the health care method.

The team exhibited moderately high aerobic (51.9 ml/kg/min.) and anaerobic (119.6 kg. meter / sec.) power, both values being significantly higher than college norms relative body fatness (89%) and a balanced mesomorphic somatotype (2.1-4.5-2.1) wherecomparable to those of athletes in other high level team sports. The structural and functional measures taken for this study appeared to indicate that the Kuwaiti team head appropriate potential for world cup. Excessively high state and trait anxiety and anger indicate that more psychological preparation was needed.

Bharshankar et. al. (2003) conducted the study to examine the effect of Yoga on cardiovascular function in subjects above 40 years of age, pulse rate, systolic and diastolic blood pressure and vise-versa ratio were studied in 50 control subjects (not doing any type of physical exercise) and 50 study subjects who had been prenticing yoga for 5 years. From the study it was observed that significant reduction in the pulse rate occurs in subjects practicing yoga (P<0.001). The difference in the mean values study group and control group was also statistically significant (P<0.01 and P<0.001) respectively.

The systolic and diastolic blood pressure showed significant positive correlation with age in the study group (r1 systolic= 0.631 and r1 diastolic = 0.610) as well as in the control group (r2 systolic = 0.981 and r2 = 0.864). The significance of difference between correlation coefficient of both the group was also tested with the use of Z transformation and the difference was significant (Z systolic = 4.041 and Z diastolic = 2.901) vise-versa ratio was also found to be significantly higher in Yoga practitioners than in controls (P<0.001).Our results indicate that yoga reduces the age related deterioration in cardio vascular functions.

The Psychological Skills Inventory for Sports (PSIS) to 149 male and 66 female collegiate rodeo athletes and performed multivariate analysis of variance (MANOVA) by event, gender, nature of competition (contact, noncontact), and athletic skills level. Psychological constructs identified by the PSIS included anxiety management, concentration, confidence, mental preparation, motivation, and team emphasis. Wilkes's criterion indicated to significant differences in psychological skills across events. Male's scores significantly higher in anxiety management, concentration, and confidence than did females. The highly skilled Ss' scoresindicated significantly higher in anxiety management, concentration, confidence, and motivation than did lower skilled Ss. Collegiate rodeo athletes exhibit psychological skills patterns inconsistent psychological skills may enhance predictions of athletic potential in this sports.

Church (2007) examined the effect of 50 percent, 100 percent, and 150 percent of the NIH Consensus Panel physical activity recommendations on cardio respiratory fitness in sedentary, overweight or obese postmenopausal women with elevated blood pressure. The Panel recommends at least 30 minutes of moderate-intensity physical activity on most, preferably all, days of the week. The study included 464 sedentary, postmenopausal overweight or obese women body mass index ranged from 25.0 to 43.0 and whose systolic blood pressure ranged from 120.0 to 159.9 mm Hg. The enrollment took place from April 2001 to June 2005.

Participants were randomly assigned to 1 of 4 energy-expenditure groups for the 6-month intervention period:

- 102 to the non-exercise control group,
- 155 to the 4-kcal/kg (400 calories) per week
- 104 to the 8-kcal/kg (800 calories) per week, and
- 103 to the 12-kcal/kg (1,200 calories) per week

The average minutes of exercising per week 72.2 for the 4-kcal/kg, 135.8 for the 8-kcal/kg, and 191.7 for the 12-kcal/kg per week exercise groups. Compared with the control group, the VO2abs (absolute) increased by 4.2 percent in the 4-kcal/kg, 6.0 percent in the 8-kcal/kg, and 8.2 percent in the 12-kcal/kg per week groups. There were no significant changes in systolic or diastolic blood pressure values from baseline to 6 months in any of the exercise groups vs. the control group. There were no substantial changes in many of the CVD risk factors or weight.

Furthermore, it was observed no changes in weight or body fat percentage, which was expected because this study was not a weight loss trial and participants were frequently informed that the objective was not weight loss and were encouraged to keep other lifestyle habits consistent from baseline throughout the study.

However, it was observed a decrease in waist circumference. It is well documented that exercise without dietary intervention has limited effectiveness in producing substantial weight loss. This may be succinctly summarized for patients and clinicians as even a little is good; more may be better.

Denis(1995)reported his findings in an indexed journal for Medicine. Theresearch paper provides a critical review of research on mental practice, with special emphasis on works investigating the role of visual imagery in this type of learning technique. Relevant   properties of images   and conditions required for their effectiveness in mental practice of motor skills are analyzed in the light of empirical evidence. The paper examines the specific question of individual imagery differences in mental practice research. Finally, implications for future research are discussed as regards the impact of certain kinds of physical training on mental imagery

Bull and Shambrook(1991) projected a concept that employing   the knowledge   we have of imagery use and the recommendations advanced regarding the delivery of a psychological skills training program, it is now more possible than ever to design imagery training programmes tailoredto meet the individual needs of developing athletes. Various approaches can be employed to teach athletes how to use psychological skills. One common approach when dealing with a number of athletes (e.g., a team) is to deliver a workshop (Bull, 1991; Brewer & Shillinglaw, 1992; Gould et al., 1990). But, how effective is a workshop for teaching athletes the values and benefits of using mental imagery, as well as showing them how to use imagery more effectively?

It was attempted to examine this question in the present study while adopting the recommendations made for providing athletes with a program individualized in terms of content and adherence-related strategies. Therefore, the purpose of this study was to investigate the influence of an imagery workshop on athletes' subsequent use of imagery. It was hypothesized that the workshop would lead to an overall increase in imagery use, and more structured and regular imagery practice.

Rushall and Lippman (1997) explored that mental practice is a recognized and often effective method for influencing the proficiency of physical performance. It is suggested, however, that "mental practice" and "imagery" are general labels applied to a variety of procedures that have different goals and uses for influencing human physical performance. This commentary argues that imagery usually is implemented for two different intentions in physical performance endeavors--skill development/learning and competition performance preparation--and those different procedures and elements are associated with each purpose. It is suggested that separation of these two functions will aid interpretation of the research and identification of issues that need empirical clarification.

Trogdon (1996)conducted a study on mental imagery and the development of pitching accuracy. The purpose of the study was determining the effect of mental imagery practice upon the improvement of pitching skills. The sample used in this study consisted of 46 male volunteers students who were registered at south-west Baptist University. The subjects were divided in to three groups by using a table of random numbers. The three methods of practice were as follows; group A, Physical Practice, group B, Mental Imagery Practice and group C, Physical Practice, and Mental Imagery Practice. A pre- test was given to the subjects prior to the experiment.

For the next four weeks subjects participated in their prescribed practice routine. The subjects threw sixty throws in each practice session and totaled 480 throws. The necessary devices were a four by six foot canvas with an area simulating a strike zone on a better. A Post-test followed the four week training period. The main gain scores for each set and each group were calculated and subjected to the dependent t-test to see if significant changes has occurred at 0.05 level. Also, an analysis of variance was computed to determine if any changes had occurred from post-test between the groups at the 0.05 level.

The result of the study indicated that all three practice groups made significant improvement between the Pre-test and Post-test scores at the 0.05 level. However, the analysis of variance yield data that found on group-B, significantly superior to the other groups.

In conclusions, the result of this study support earlier research which indicates the use of mental imagery will improve the performance of a physical skill, Subjects who followed their accuracy scores as well as those combined Physical and Mental Practice. While some of the practice modes proved to be superior to the others, a positive statement could be made for the use of mental imagery in that the physical practice group showed no superiority.

Smith(1997) conducted a study on evaluation of an imagery training programme with intercollegiate basketball players. The purpose of this study was to develop an imagery training programme using the best procedures currently known and b) to evaluate this imagery training in a real life or field setting. It was conducted over an entire competitive season using the University of Illinois men's basketball team as the treatment group and two other conference teams as the treatment group and two other conference teams as control groups. Changes in

33

physical and psychology skill were measured primarily through case studies utilizing inventories and observation.

Evaluation of the imagery training programme was accomplished by answering 4 target questions: 1) Does imagery training provide the athletes with increased ability for reducing competitive anxiety? 2) Does imagery training improve self-confidence over time in specific area like shooting and ball handling? 3) Does imagery training improve the execution of specific strategies like offensive and defensive execution? 4) Does imagery training improve overall basketball performance? Various inventories and recording logs were used to answer each of these questions.

Both inferential and descriptive statistics were used for data analysis. For the Sport Competitive Anxiety Test (SCAT), imagery in sport, and coaches' questionnaire administered pre and post session to the treatment and control groups; an analysis of covariance design was used with the pre-season measure as the covariate. For the few questions with only 2 or 3 possible answers a chi-square analysis was used to determine differences between the treatment and control groups. For the pre competitive CSAI-2 inventory, the baseline measure was covariate.

Answer to each of the target questions were as follows:

1) It cannot be concluded that the imagery training programme decreased competitive state anxiety because the Illinois and control groups showed no differences of their competitive state anxiety measures and no consistent trend among the case studies was evident in this area. 2) A variety of evidence suggests that imagery training may have improved self-confidence in specific areas shooting

and ball handling in individual cases, but weight of the evidence remains inconclusive. 3) The imagery training improves the specific strategies like offensive and defensive execution. 4) The case studies indicated that the athletes who developed commitment to the imagery training tended to believe that the programme improved their basketball performance.

Fahleson(1986) investigated the effect of teaching acts on the thoughts and performance of fourth, sixth and eighth grade students. When learning a novel Jai AlaiLike (Scoop ball). Three intact elementary physical education classes at the University of Wyoming preparatory school were used as subject in the study. Prior to administration of the instructional treatments, students completed questionnaires and tests assessing their imagery ability (Kinesthetic or Visual), Anxiety, and the skill ability on the scoop ball task.

Structured lessons in the scoop ball task were scripted and presented using cues (minding) and information that prompted students to think about their performance in either visual or kinesthetic ways. All students received both of the instructional treatments. Performance in the scoop ball skill was measured on an objective, low-inference skill test. Students were being briefed following instruction using a stimulated recall procedure.

This investigation assessed the main effect of aptitudes and treatments; assessed aptitude treatment interactions and examined students' cognitive processes there was no performance difference between the two imagery performance groups. There was a significant (P< .05) perceived treatment X initial ability interaction perceived treatment X initial ability interaction. Perceived kinesthetic instruction was associated with higher posttest scored for persons scoring low on the pretest and pretest and visual instruction was associated with higher post test scores for highly skilled subjects. Those student who reported remembering using, and finding the minding helpful were the poorer performance, but they rated their performance higher than those who reported not remembering, using of finding the minding helpful.

The result of this study show that the students regularly think about instruction in way different from those the teacher intended. It was found that effective minding are vivid and image evoking and students have preferred ways of imaging movement that are the result of meta cognitive decisions rather than designed instruction.

Burstein(1986) conducted a study on the effect of using video imagery fusion in learning swimming skills. In this study, thirty volunteer college students were rated by six expert judges on their performance in an out of water swimming technique. The subjects were divided equally in to a traditional mental practice group, a control group and a video-imagery fusion (VIF) group. Each subject was videotaped on his/her out of water technique at the beginning, middle and conclusion of the 3/1/2 week experiments period. Kendall's Coefficient of Concordance showed a high degree of inter – rate reliability and yield the scores for each subject used in the statistical analysis. A MANCOVA procedure with a repeated measures design showed a significant (P<.05) improvement for all groups from the mid test to the post test using the pre test scores as the covariant measures.

The VIF group improved mostly during the first half of the training period. The traditional mental practice group showed its greatest improvement during the first half of the experiments period and the control group improve throughout the training period. The use of VIF as a mental practice improves throughout the training period. The use of VIF as a mental practice technique or recovery faces of the crawl stroke, but not necessary more effective other than methods of learning.

Hough (1995) investigated the effect of varying imagery perspective and imagery time on performance of the putting stroke in golf. A series of audio tapes developed for the research, served as the psychological skills training programme (PSTP). Subjects in the experimental groups (n=28) were from 3 introductory golf classes. The control group (n=7) was from the general student population. Subjects were randomly assigned to 1 to 4 treatments groups of 7 subjects per group. The 4 group were the internal perspective 3 minute imagery group, the external perspective 3 minute imagery group the internal perspective 7 minute imagery group.The three dependent variables were 20 scores (10 pre and posttest) on putting trials control of visual imagery measured by the Gorden test or visual imagery control (TVIC), and vividness of mental imagery measured by the Betts questionnaire upon mental imagery vividness (QUMIV).

All groups were pre and post tested following an interval of 6 week treatment period. All groups performed a putting activity once each week during the 6 week treatment period. The treatment subjects listened to audio tapes three times each week during the treatment period. The control group did not listen to the audio tapes.

The following are conclusions based upon the hypothesis, statistical findings, limitations and delimitations of the study:

(1) The rejection of the null hypothesis of the treatment effects on groups 2, 3 and 5 suggests that, for 3 and 7 minute internal groups and the 7 minute external group, improvement in their putting ability is due to the treatment conditions, group

4 (the 3 minute external group) did show improvement but not at a statistically significant level.

(2) The rejection of the null hypotheses on the repeated measures pre and post tests for putting, TVIC and QUMIV scores, for all groups including controls, suggests that improvement may have been a result of putting practice and the desire to improve due to involvement in the study as well as the treatment. Participation in the study and putting practice were associated with increase in putting and imagery ability by the control group as well as the treatment group.

Szabo Attila et. al. (1994) examined the association between maximal aerobic power (VO-sub(Zmax)) and blood pressure (BP) and heart rate (HR) reactivity to mental challenge. 20 adolescent male judo athletes (aged 14-17 Years) performed a 2-min mental arithmetic task. BP in the immediate stress-recovery period was not related to VO-sub(2max), but Ss' having a higher VO-sub(2max) showed faster HR recovery from mental stress than did those having a lower VO-sub(2max). Ss' who showed earlier peak HR responses during the stress episode demonstrated lower average HR reactivity than did Ss' who attained the maximal HR responses later in the stress period.

Overby (1996) investigated this study to ascertain whether or not a relationship exists between dance experience, imagery ability and body awareness. Twenty experienced female dancers 18-30 years of age (with five or more years of dance training), and twenty novice female dancers 18-30 years of age (with one year of less of dance training), were utilized. Each subject performed two body awareness tasks and computed four imagery questionnaires. The Directionally (D) body awareness task required that the subject move in a specific floor pattern, direction, and spatial orientation.

The Reflective Body Perception (R) body awareness task required the subjects to accurately reproduce body position. In both tasks the subjects viewed the criterion movement on a large screen video monitor and were then videotaped as they reproduced the movement satisfaction (SAMS) (Nelson and Allen, 1970). This body image test measured the image the subject has to herself as moving entity. The second questionnaire, the Movement Imagery Questionnaire (MIQ) (Hall and Pongrace, 1983), measured individual differences in visual and kinesthetic imagery of movements. The third imagery questionnaire, the Individual Differences Questionnaire (IDQ), (Paivio, 1970 measured the degree to which a subject habitually used imaginal or verbal modes of thinking.

The fourth questionnaire, Stumps Cube Test (SCT) (Stumpt, 1980), measured visuo-spatial ability. A MANOVA 2x2x2 (experience x task x sight) with repeated measured on the last two factors, revealed that the body awareness (D and R) was significantly better in experienced dancers than in novice dancers. Hotteling's revealed that experienced dancers differed significantly from novice dancers. On three if the imagery ability measured (SAMS, IDO, and SCT) and revealed no significant correlation between novice and experienced dancer's body awareness and imagery ability. All subjects reported using imaginable strategies to enhance their ability to reproduce the criterion movements. This study supported the contention that a relationship exists between dance experience imagery ability, and body awareness.

Stall, Beckett, Mclean and Lusquellac(1990) conducted a study on mental training in the pool they institute a comprehensive mental training program for a team college swimmers (N=50) and divers (N=6). This program was to address several areas including performance anxiety, cognitive processes, and performance consequences of mental skills training. In conjunction with the coaches and athletes, a sport psychologist assisted in the formulation of goals and objectives. The training techniques consisted of relaxation, concentration imagery, positive mental attitude, cognitive relaxation, and creative problem solving.

Relaxation and concentration exercise were emphasized as precursors to the incorporation of the other techniques. Groups were joined to participated in join 45 minute guided relaxation of imagery sessions ever 2 day, with emphasis placed on the athlete's ability to self-induce the same states. The athletes and coaches then implemented regular used of the techniques. The results showed the program was successful with enhancement of both cognitive state (such as confidence and motivation) and physical best during the swimmers and drivers session as compared to the previous seasons.

Veddli(1992) conducted a study on the "Effect of Mental Practice and Interaction of Perceptual Style of Elementary Grade Level on Performance of Coincidence Anticipation Motor Task". The purpose of his study was to determine the effectiveness of mental practice as a teaching methodology and the interaction of perceptual style with this methodology at three elementary grade level (two, four, and six). The dependent variable was the accuracy of the performance of each S N=144) on the final tail of a coincidence-anticipation motor task (C/A- Skill).

Barton et al. (1996) used sports and sports type as a vehicle for examining attributions for success / failure pride and anxiety of 111 college aged 17-25 years athletes. It was shown that both individual team sport athletes and team sport athletes differ little in their emotional reactions and attributions to outcome. Internal and external attributions were shown to be two separate factors. Experienced college-aged athletes exhibited both high internality and high externality for success and both internality and low externality for failure. As expected, level of pride was found to be greater for success than failure. Greater anxiety occurred after failure than success, but post competition anxiety reactions were shown to be attribution independent emotions.

Previous research on self-serving, self-enhancing and self-protecting biases was found to be inadequate in explaining the intricacies and diversity of attributional responses present in this field study. It is suggested that differences in findings across studies regarding attributional biasness may be based on the methodologies and instruments used, limitations on the number of attributions available to subjects, differences between subject populations tested, the way in which researchers conceive of attributional findings and finally the way in which attributions are defined. The findings lend support to the cognition or 'information processing' theoretical viewpoint.

Filaire et. al. (2001) the study aimed to investigate the salivary testosterone (T) and cortisol (C) and the mental state responses to a real football championship among 18 male competitors (mean age 22.2 years). Data about individual's anxiety levels, strategies of coping, and patterns of behavior were thus collected. The relationship between hormonal changes and psychological variables were also analyzed. Results showed C responses to competition, which was especially characterized by an anticipatory rise. Depending on outcome, results did not show significantly different C responses. The T values noted after the last fight were significantly greater in the losers than those obtained in the winners. Hormonal response did not show a relationship with psychological variables depending on the outcome. Losers showed just before the first fight an elevated cognitive anxiety, accompanied by low self-confidence.

Ahern and Lochr (1996) in the study, it was found that that thepsychosocial factors increasingly are becoming recognized as significant factors in sports performance, injury prevention, rehabilitation, and management, whichclearly indicates about the successful performance in any sport—for example, basketball—requires the athlete to possess the necessary physical abilities, talent, and fundamental skills, such as: speed, ball handling, passing, and shooting. Whether considering an individual or team sport, however, the contribution of focused attention, concentration, stress management, and cognitive strategies is important.

In most sports, athletes and coaches alike commonly refer to the "mental game" as equally important as physical abilities and talent to overall performance. Indeed, for the elite and professional athlete, the mental game often provides the competitive edge necessary for winning.

This article presents an overview of the psychosocial and behavioral risk factors known to contribute to sports injury risk and rehabilitation. Space limitations obviously preclude a detailed examination of all aspects of psychosocial assessment and intervention for sports injury. Nevertheless, the major approaches are presented and described with sufficient detail to assist the sports medicine practitioner in evaluating and considering the potential value of this approach in his or her practice. For the interested reader, more detail about a particular technique or procedure can be found through the reference material.

Ursuliak et. al. (2003) conducted a research with the goals of this work were to assess the effects of participation in mindfulness meditation-based stress reduction program on mood disturbance and symptoms of stress in cancer outpatients immediately after and 6 months after program completion. A convenience sample of eligible cancer patients were enrolled after they had given informed consent. All patients completed the Profile of Mood States (POMS) and Symptoms of Stress Inventory (SOSI) both before and after the intervention and 6 months later. The intervention consisted of a mindfulness meditation group lasting 1.5 h each week for 7 weeks, plus daily home meditation practice.

A total of 89 patients, average age 51, provided pre-intervention data. Eighty patients provided post intervention data and 54 completed the 6-month follow-up. The participants were heterogeneous with respect to type and stage of cancer. Patients' scores decreased significantly from before to after the intervention on the POMS and SOSI total scores and most subscales, indicating less mood disturbance and fewer symptoms of stress, and these improvements were maintained at the 6-month follow-up.

More advanced stages of cancer were associated with less initial mood disturbance, while more home practice and higher initial POMS scores predicted improvements on the POMS between the pre- and post-intervention scores. Female gender and more education were associated with higher initial

The SOSI scores and improvements on the SOSI were predicted by more education and greater initial mood disturbance. This program was effective in decreasing mood disturbance and stress symptoms for up to 6 months in both male and female patients with a wide variety of cancer diagnoses, stages of illness, and educational background, and with disparate ages.

In a study conducted by Boon (1977) the relationship of arousal and anxiety with gymnastic performance was investigated. Pulse rate and palmer sweating were utilized as indicants of arousal. Anxiety was assessed by means of the State-Trait Anxiety Inventory. The Ithaca college women's varsity gymnastic team (N=18) was tested during the1973-74 Season. The inter-correlation matrix of all variables, pulse rate, palmer sweating, state anxiety, trait anxiety and gymnastic performance revealed limited relationships between gymnastic performance and arousal/anxiety measures.

Klavora (1975) studied optimal pre-competitive state anxiety of football players. Oxidine's proposition regarding the optimal arousal level for the typical participant in football was examined on 4 level of football competition: Junior High School, Senior High School, Alberta Junior and University. The pre-competitive state anxiety was measured by Spielberger's STAI anxiety scale. No Significant differences in optimal pre-competitive state anxiety at the competitive levels were found.

Greenblatt, S. Shavasana (1999) mindfulness-based Stress Reduction (MBSR) is an 8-week clinical intervention developed by Kabat-Zinn and colleagues in the 1970s and 1980s. Mindfulness meditation is the key component of MBSR, and patients are typically asked to meditate 45 minutes daily. The present study aimed to assess the directionality of the relationship between meditation and stress. This was done with path analysis. The study also examined stress reactivity's role in meditation's healthful effects. Finally, the study assessed the relative importance of different aspects of meditation practice, including length and frequency of meditation.

The sample included 180 persons practicing meditation similar to mindfulness meditation, recruited from meditation centers around the U.S. Subjects completed self-report measures on meditation habits, the Weekly Stress Inventory (WSI), and the Short Form-36V health survey. To assess causality between meditation and stress reactivity, the WSI and the meditation questionnaire were re-administered two weeks after initial data collection. Data were collected primarily via the internet. The first path analysis compared two models differing only on the causal direction of the path between stress reactivity and recent meditation. The

44

model positing recent meditation influencing stress reactivity provided a better fit to the data than the model positing stress reactivity influencing meditation practice. The second analysis examined the path coefficients of a similar but fully identified model. This also showed meditation's influence on stress reactivity to provide a better fit to the data than the alternative model.

A strong negative association was found between stress reactivity and health. Also, frequency of meditation was as important to stress reactivity as hours meditated. Additionally, when examining the differential importance of recent meditation vs. lifetime meditation experience, recent meditation was associated with emotional health, vitality, and stress reactivity, whereas lifetime meditation experience was relatively unimportant. This study has some implications for MBSR, including the importance of continued meditation practice after patients complete MBSR. Another such implication concerns the equal importance of frequency of meditation vs. length of meditation sessions. This study is an initial effort at addressing the role of stress reactivity in meditation's effects. Further efforts studying these phenomena with clinical populations are needed.

Telama and Silvennoinen (1999) conducted a study with a purposeto assess the reasons young adults participate in physical exercise and leisure-time physical activity. The MPAQ contains 33 items focusing on the conscious reflection of physical activity interests, the advance planning of physical activities, and the influence of weather and friends on one's own physical activities. Individuals respond using a 3-point ordinal scale. Previous empirical research on motivation for physical activity was drawn upon in constructing the items and measurement methods. Physical component factor analysis (n=3106) followed by varimax rotation supported an eight-factor solution accounting for 21.3% of the variance.

45

The factors were labeled as Fitness Related to the Self Image, Relaxation, Sociability, Preference for Outdoor Activities, Normative Health, Competition and Achievement, Improving One's Physique and Functional Health. Psychometric data were reported for 3,106 students residing in Finland. These students were selected through stratified-random bluster sampling and represented grades 2-3, 5-6 and 8-9.

Otsuki T. et al. (2007) studied to investigate whether post exercise HR recovery accelerates in strength-trained athletes. Subjects were young strength trained athletes (ST. N =12) endurance trained athletes (ET: N=12), and age matched sedentary control men (C; N=12) HR and oxygen uptake were measured during submaximal exercise (cycling exercise, 40% maximal oxygen uptake for 8 min) and 30sec. after the exercise (the post exercise period) The results suggest that the HR recovery immediately after exercise is accelerated in both strength and endurance trained athletes.

Pfeiffer, K.A., et al. (2007) studied to determine how factors are related to change in cardiorespiratory fitness across time in middle school girls followed through high school Adolescent girls (N=274, 59% African American, Baseline age = 13.6+0.6 years) performed a submaximal fitness test in 8th, 9th, and 12th grades. Height, weight, sports participation, and physical activity were also measured. Moderate-to-vigorous physical activity and vigorous physical activity were determined by the number of blocks reported on the 3 day physical Activity Recall. Individual differences and developmental change in CRF were assessed simultaneously by calculating individual growth curves for each participant using growth curve modeling.

Although there were fluctuations in PWC170 Scores across time, average scores decreased during 4 yr. Physical activity was related to change in CRF over time; BMI race and sport participation were also important factors related to change over time in CRF (depending on expression of CRF-weight relative V/s absolute) Subsequent research should focus on explaining the complex interaction between CRF.

Rowlands, et al. (2007) studied to determine the relationship of tri-axial accelerometry, uniaxial accelerometry and pedometry with speed and step frequency across a range of walking and running speeds. Nine male runners wore two ActiGraph uniaxial accelerometer and pedometry with speed and step frequency across a range of walking and running speeds. Nine male runners wore two ActiGraph Uniaxial accelerometers. Two RT3 tri-axial accelerometer (all set at a 1-s epoch) and two pedometers. Each participant walked 60 S. at 4 and 6 Kmh. ran for 60 s at 10, 12, 14, 16, and 18 Kmh-1, and ran for 30 s at 20 22, 24, and 26 Kmh-1 Step frequency was recorded by a visual count.

It was concluded that increasing underestimation of activity by the ActiGraph as speed increases is related to frequency dependent filtering and assessment of acceleration in the vertical place only. RT3 vector magnitude was strongly related to speed, reflecting the predominance of horizontal acceleration at higher speeds. These results indicate that high intensity activity is underestimated by the ActiGraph even after correction for frequency dependent filtering, but not by the RT3 Pedometer output is highly correlated with step frequency.

Huang et al. (2007) studied to evaluate the cross sectional relationship between BMI and physical fitness index (PFI) based on four indicators of fitness in a national sample of Taiwanese youth. Height weight, and four measures of physical fitness (sit-ups completed in 60 s. standing long jump, sit and reach, and 800 or 1600m run walk) were measured in a national sample of 102.75 Taiwanese youth 9-18 years of age 50.940 girls and 51.825 boys.

It was concluded that declines in a curvilinear manner with increasing BMI among youth 9-18 yr. of age, but the slope of the relationship varies with age. Takeshima also studied to compare the effects of aerobic, resistance, flexibility, balance, and Taj-chi programs of FF in Japanese older adults. FF was evaluated using a chair stand arm curl, up and go, sit and reach back scratch, functional reach, and 12 minutes' walk one hundred thirteen older adults (73+6 years, 64 men, 49 women) concluded that results suggest that a single mode with crossover effects could address multiple components of fitness. Therefore, a well-rounded exercise program may only need to consist of two types of exercise to improve the components of functional fitness one type should be aerobic exercise, and the second type could be chosen from RES, BAL and T-CHI.

Shah, Singh and Pathak (1990) administered personality questionnaire and competitive state inventory-2 on twenty one international marathon runners to investigate extraversion, neuroticism, psychotism and state anxiety, cognitive anxiety, self-confidence. The result obtained indicated that successful marathon runners found to have high mean value in age (chronological) extraversion, neuroticism and self-confidence scale, where as low mean value in psychotism, cognitive anxiety, somatic anxiety and total competitive state anxiety.

Castelli et al. (2007) studied physical fitness and academic achievement in third -and fifth grade students. The relationship between physical fitness and academic achievement has received much attention owing to the increasing prevalence of children who are overweight and unfit, as well as the inescapable pressure on schools to produce students who meet academic standards. This study examined 259 public school students in third and fifth grades and found that filed tests of physical fitness were positively related to academic achievement.

Specifically aerobic capacity was positively associated with achievement, whereas BMI was inversely related. Associations were demonstrated in total academic achievement, mathematics achievement and reading achievement thus suggesting that aspect of physical fitness may be globally related to academic performance in preadolescents. His findings are discussed with regards to maximizing school performance and the implications for educational policies.

Physical fitness and Anthropometrical profile of the Brazilian Male Judo Team. The present study had as objectives (1) to compare the morphological and functional characteristics of the male judo players of the Brazilian Team (A (n=7) with the judo players of Teams B and C (reserves: n=15), and (20 to verify the association between the variables measured. Thus, 22 athletes from the seven Olympic weight categories were submitted to : a body composition evaluation (Body mass, height, ten skinfolds, eight circumferences, three bone diameters and percent body fat estimation); the special Judo Fitness Test (SJFT); maximal strength tests (one repetition- maximum, 1 RM, in bench press, row, and squat) and the Cooper test. One-way analysis of covariance was used to compare the groups.

The relationships between variables were determined by the Pearson coefficient correlation. The significance level was fixed at 5% No. significant difference was found in any variable between them. The main significant correlations observed were between the following variables VO2 max and number of throws in the SJFT (r= 0.79) percent body fat and estimated VO2 max (r= -0.83) and number of throws in the SJFT (r=-0.70); chest circumference and bench press

1 RM (r=0.90) and in the row (r=0; 86). However, there was no significant correlation between circumferences and I RM/kg of body mass.

According to these results the main conclusion are: (1) the physical variables measured do not discriminate performance when analysis is directed to the best athletes: (2) a higher percent body fat is negatively correlated with performance in activities with body mass locomotion (Cooper test and the SJFT); (3) Judo players with higher aerobic power performed better in high-intensity intermittent exercise; (4) Judo players with bigger circumferences present bigger absolute maximal strength.

Physical fitness was measured by a maximal treadmill exercise test. Average follow-up was slightly more than 8 years, for a total of 110 482 person-years of observation. There were 240 deaths in men and 43 deaths in women. Age-adjusted all-cause mortality rates declined across physical fitness quintiles from 64.0 per 10 000 person-years in the least-fit men to 18.6 per 10 000 person-years in the most-fit men (slope, -4.5). Corresponding values for women were 39.5 per 10 000 person-years to 8.5 per 10 000 person-years (slope, -5.5).

These trends remained after statistical adjustment for age, smoking habit, cholesterol level, systolic blood pressure, fasting blood glucose level, parental history of coronary heart disease, and follow-up interval. Lower mortality rates in higher fitness categories also were seen for cardiovascular disease and cancer of combined sites. Attributable risk estimates for all-cause mortality indicated that low physical fitness was an important risk factor in both men and women. Higher levels of physical fitness appear to delay all-cause mortality primarily due to lowered rates of cardiovascular disease and cancer.

The purpose of the study was to compare the performances of entering Filipino freshman students at the University of the Philippines and American and Japanese boys in the AAHPER Youth Fitness Test. Four age classifications (15, 16, 17 and 18 years and above) were included in the study.

Significant differences in performances were determined through the application of the chi-square test of significance. The statistical method was used to analyze the distribution of Filipino boys and the quartile limits of the American and Japanese norms for the Youth Fitness test

The findings showed that American and Japanese boys performed better in more items of the Youth Fitness Test than the Filipino students. This was true for all age groups, with the exception of the 15 year-old Filipino boys who performed better than their American counterparts. The Filipinos performed poorly in the sit-up and softball throw, but, they excelled in the shuttle run.

Physical fitness, participation in physical activity, fundamental motor skills and body composition are important contributors to the health and the development of a healthy lifestyle among children and youth. The New South Wales Schools Fitness and Physical Activity Survey, 1997, was conducted to fill some of the gaps in our knowledge of these aspects of the lives of young people in New South Wales. The survey was conducted in February and March, 1997 and collected data on a randomly-selected sample of students (n = 5518) in Years 2, 4, 6, 8 and 10.

Measures were taken on body composition (height and weight, waist and hip girths, skinfolds), health-related fitness (aerobic capacity, muscular strength, muscular endurance, flexibility), fundamental motor skills (run, vertical jump, catch, overhand throw, forehand strike and kick), self-reported physical activity, time spent

51

in sedentary recreation, and physical education (PE) classes. The methods are described to assist in the development of surveys of other populations and to provoke debate relevant to the development and dissemination of standard approaches to monitoring the fitness, physical activity habits and body composition of Australian children and youth. Finally, we offer comments on some of the strengths and limitations of the methods employed.

Singh et. al. (1986) studied the anxiety difference between male and female handball players of intervarsity level. 73 (male 36, female 37) subjects comprising 6 teams were investigated. The subjects were members of 1st, 2nd and 3rd position holders respectively. Marten's sports competitive anxiety test (SCAT) for adults was administered to the subjects selected or the study. T test was applied to find out intra group differences. ANOVA was worked out to find out the difference among the different position holder of male and female teams. The difference of competitive anxiety between male and female came out to be statistically significant at .05 level though over all level is moderate in both cases.

Zwart (1987) studied attention and anxiety responses of athletes to mental tainting technique. This study explores the change in competition anxiety, attention direction and focus, and performance in 13-15 year old swimmer (n=30) after exposure to the super learning mental training program. The experimental treatment consisted of engaging the subjects in a six weak (two hour session per weak) program of (i) relaxation training, (ii) positive affirmation statements synchronized to breathing exercises and music, and (iii) visualization for mental rehearsal.

Allen (1993) conducted the study on the effect of mental practice and physical practice of the improvement of golf swing. The purpose of this study was to determine the effects of mental practice and physical practice on the improvement of golf swing. The modified Benson 5 – Iron test was used to measure distance and accuracy or each subject.

The study utilized 40 numerical male and females class room volunteers form physical education class at the University of 'Mississippi'. This was a four group designed using analysis of variances and a pre-test consisted of testing subjects using a modified Benson 5- Iron test for distance and accuracy. Measurement for distance and accuracy were obtained in the same manner by testing subject using the modified the Benson 5- Iron test.

Singh (1987) administered SCAT (Marten`s) to Indian athletes and hockey players and found significant differences between the two samples on sport competition anxiety. Hockey players, both male and female, were found to have less competition anxiety as compared with the players of individual events. Males exhibited less anxiety in competitive situations as compared with the females.

Radha (1995) studied the selected psychological variable namely anxiety aggression, motivation and personality traits in relation to basketball performance. If psychological factors, aggression is highly correlated with the playing ability (r = .941) further, it is noted that the coefficient of multiple correlation (r = .981) revealed that psychological factor put together play an important role in the basketball performance.

Weinberg (1980) investigated the relationship between competition trait anxiety and state anxiety and golf performance in a field setting. Test low moderate and high CTA collegiate golfer (10 per cell) performed in a practice round one day and day 2 of competitive tournament. Co-relation between SCAT and state anxiety indicated that SCAT was good predicator of pre-competitive state anxiety. The direction of state anxiety and performance CTA main effects provide support for oxedine`s (1970) contentions that requiring fine muscle coordination and precision (i.g. golf) are performed best at low level of anxiety.

Morgan (1970) administered three forms of IPAT 8- parallel form anxiety test to seven varsity wrestlers at the University of Missouri. The first test was given before the season began, a second 45-60 minutes prior to a match judged easy by the coach. Surprisingly the pre-match anxiety scores were lower than the pre-season scores, but there was no difference in anxiety scores between the easy and difficult matches.

Marten (1982) study conducted on four sample of Volleyball team found subjects scoring high on Achievement Motivation (Mehrabian Scale) are low in fear of failure and high in need achievement. Same way subjects scoring low on Achievement Motivation Scale were found high in fear of failure and low in motive to success. The study further concluded that there was no significant relationship between sports competition anxiety and achievement motivation.

Carder (1966) found the relationship between manifest anxiety and performance in college football. The subjects were 40 freshman football players who were rated on 2 scales by 3 members of the coaching staff. One scale consisted of ranking on total performance during the season and the other scale involved skill rating in blocking, tackling, movement agility, and running speed. Subjects were also tested on the M.A.S. and 3 motor ability tests to identify potential. The results indicated no significant relationships between the M.A.S. Scores and total performance, individual skill performance, or actualization of football potential.

Silva (1981) tried to identify variable that are related to optimal performance at elite levels of wrestling. The subjects were 86 candidates competing for 1980 US Greco-Roman and free style Olympic wrestling teams. Psychological testing included trait testing and pre-competitive state testing. The reports showed non-qualifier scored higher than qualifiers on anxiety, depression and regression. Separate anxiety measures generated from the STAI and the IPAT anxiety trait measures indicated that the qualifiers were lower on all measures of anxiety than were the non-qualifiers.

Harris (1964) compared high and low fitness indices college women in Psychological traits and found that there is a tendency for the 'fit' individual to appear more stable in certain Psychological traits and to appear less anxious in others.

Dowthwaity (1984) administered Spielberger's State and Trait Anxiety Inventory and SCAT to 22 women hockey players. Forwards reported consistently higher A-State than defenders. Consistent differences in A-State Score were found in the 1st XIth for the extreme group of high and low score on SCAT and the high SCAT group showed the greater increase from the coaching to the competitive condition. Over both teams A-State correlated significantly with SCAT.

A study conducted by Goodspeed (1984) investigated the effects of comprehensive self-regulation training including relaxation, mental imagery, self-confidence, concentration and cognitive restructuring on anxiety and performance of female gymnasts.

Griffith, Steel and Vaccaro (1999) examined the relationship between the anxiety level and performance of 62 beginning Scuba diving students and standardization that there was no relationship between anxiety and performance on relatively simple cost, while there was a relationship between anxiety and performance on the more complex diving maneuvers.

Purpose of the study conducted by Sandhu et al. (1986) was to adapt the competitive anxiety level scale for female basketball players. 32 female basketball players were taken as subjects from the basketball teams of colleges officiated to PunjabUniversity. The data were statistically analyzed by using the statistical operation including co-efficient or correlation to determine the validity. Factor analysis was also used for the adaptation of test. The result of the study revealed that the test is valid and can be used on female basketball players at college level in Indian conditions.

Baker (1962) studied the effects of anxiety and stress on gross motor performance. Sixty one male students with scores more than 1S.D. above (high anxiety) and below (low anxiety) the mean on the Pittsburgh revision revision of the Manifest Anxiety Scale were used as subjects and assigned randomly in each category to experimental and control groups. The test consisted of matching a specified foot pattern while walking at 2mph on a treadmill for 1.5 minutes, with total missteps constituting the error score. The experimental groups received shock at predetermined intervals. Subject had two trials with pulse rate recorded before and after each trial. Following each trial, the subjects rated themselves on the anxiety during the test. The findings supported the hypothesis that the stress inhibited efficient function of high anxiety subject facilitated the performance.

CHAPTER - III

PROCEDURE AND METHODOLOGY

In this chapter, the research scholar explained how he has conducted the present research work. The procedure has been explained in line with the delimitations, objectives and selected variables and protocol of testing procedures. For the purpose of the present study, the applied procedure and methodology was explained, which were adopted under the following headings like: selection of the subjects, selection of the variables and their tests, design of the study, instrumental reliability, reliability of data and subjects, administration of the tests, and administration of anthropological tests, physical fitness and psychological tests items to assess the psycho-motor ability, collection of the data and statistical procedure applied for the study, have been described in details:

Selection of the Subjects:

Initially, one hundred Kabaddi and Kho-Kho players were selected on random basis for the present study. The designated delimitations for the present study were kept in mind for the selection of the subjects; those have participated in Delhi School's Zonal, Inter-zonal and School National Games represented respective team of Delhi Schools. It was also taken into consideration that all the selected subjects were ranged from 16 to 19 years of age and who were involved in regular practice for their respective games of Kabaddi and Kho-Kho to remain physically and mentally fit. Finally, total 50 players were randomly selected from Kabaddi and 50 players were selected from game of Kho-Kho. It was also kept in mind that all the subjects should participate voluntarily for purpose of data collection during present study.

Selection of the Variables and their Tests:

For the present study, the research scholar has gone through the various literatures to finalize the variables. The selection of the variables was utmost important as the total procedure and administration was dependent upon the nature of selection of variables. The variables are the key direction for the nature of the findings and outcomes from the present study. The experts were also consulted to get appropriate and rational suggestions to finalize the variables. The following variables and their test items anthropological and psycho-physical variables were selected for the purpose of present study:

Anthropological Components:
- (a) Height
- (b) Body Weight
- (c) Body Mass Index (BMI)

Physical Fitness Components and their Tests:

(a) Speed	:	40m. Sprint Test
(b) Explosive Strength	:	Standing Broad Jump
(c) Cardio-vascular Endurance	:	12min. run/walk test
(d) Coordinative Ability	:	4X10 m Shuttle Run
(e) Flexibility	:	Sit and Reach Test
(f) Muscular Strength	:	One Minute Sit-ups

Psychological Components and their Tests:

The psychological abilities were measured through the selected test items mentioned here as under:

(a) Psycho-motor Ability   : Eye-hand Coordination Test

(b) Concentration   : Grid Concentration Test

(c) Sports Competition Anxiety Test (SCAT)

Design of the Study:

The design of the study was on the basis to compare the groups specified for Kabaddi and Kho-Kho in relation to the selected variables related to psycho-motor abilities. The selected tests were administered and their measurements were for the test items such as: Height, Body Weight, Body Mass Index (BMI), Speed: 40m Sprint, Explosive Strength: Standing Broad Jump, Cardio-vascular Endurance: 12 minutes Run/Walk Test, Coordinative Ability: 4X10m Shuttle Run, Flexibility: Sit and Reach Test, Psycho-motor Ability: Eye-hand Coordination Test, Concentration: Grid Concentration Test and Sports Competition Anxiety Test (SCAT).

The tests were conducted on all the one hundred randomly and voluntarily selected subjects and data were collected. The present study was designed to assess the comparison among the selected group of players of Kabaddi and Kho-Kho. The above mentioned variables were the basis of the present study for which it was designed to collect the appropriate data from the selected test items. The appropriate statistical analyses were applied for assessing the requisite results related to Kabaddi and Kho-Kho players.

Administration of the Test Items:

The research scholar has adopted required guidelines and precautions to be followed. The prescriptions suggested by Rikli and Jones for administration of the selected test items were taken into consideration. The detailed procedures for administering different tests have been described here as under:

1. Body Mass Index*(Height and Weight):*

The Body Mass Index (BMI) is a simple measure of the lean weight and fat weight components. It is used in epidemiological research and has a moderately high correlation (r=-.69) with body density. It is easily calculated from the following formula:

$$BMI = Weight / Height^2$$

Where, the weight is measured in kilograms and height in meters.

BMI is a very simple tool. Its best use is for risk assessment for the general population to calculate body fat. It was compared to height-weight tables though; it has a much higher association with body fat of a person. It has another simple formula to calculate the BMI:

BMI = Body mass in kilograms/ (Height x Height in meters)

(Divide if weight is in lbs. by 2.2046 to get weight in kilograms)

So, as an example a 150lb (68kg) man/woman who is 165cm(1.65m) tall.

BMI = 68/ (1.65 x 1.65)

= 68/ 2.7

BMI = 25.185

This person has a Body Mass Index of 25.185 then there is an association between BMI and many major degenerative diseases. As, BMI increases so does their risk of ill health.

TABLE: 1

BODY MASS INDEX AT A GLANCE TO VIEW THE STATUS

Classification	Risk	BMI Score
Underweight	Moderate	less than 18.5
Normal	Very low	18.5 - 24.9
Overweight	Low	25.0 - 29.9
Obese Class 1	Moderate	30.0 - 34.9
Obese class 2	High	35.0 - 39.9
Extreme obesity	Very high	greater than 40.0

2. SPEED: 40M SPRINT

Purpose: To assess speed

Objective: To run as fast as possible.

Equipment: Two stopwatches, athletics track or leveled surface to run, lime powder to mark.

Instructions: For safety purposes, the subjects were asked to do warm-up for 20minutes including- jogging, strides, loosening, stretching exercises etc. They were also explained and   demonstrated sprint start and its commands.

Procedure: After a light warming-up period, the subjects took his/her position on the line. Four subjects run at a time. On signal 'GO' the subjects started his/her race.

Scoring: The score was taken as lower time of two stop watches for each subject.

3. STANDING BROAD JUMP:

Purpose: To measure Explosive power

Equipment: Measuring tape and jumping pit.

Procedure: The subject stood behind the takeoff line. He/she were asked to bend his / her backward before the execution of jump. Then he/she jumped forward by extending his/her knees and swings his/her arms forward and upward simultaneously. Measurement was taken from the heel impression closest to the takeoff line to the inner edge of the takeoff line. He/she executed take off from both the feet and jumped as ahead as possible and landed on both the feet. Three trials were permitted.

Scoring: The score was the best of the three distances recorded in feet and inches.

4. CARDIOVASCULAR ENDURANCE: 12MIN. RUN/WALK TEST:

Purpose: To assess endurance

Objective: To run/walk as fast as possible for 12 minutes

Equipment: 400m /200m Athletics Track, stop watch, track is used or another suitable running area measured so that exact distances are indicated. Distance covered in 12-minutes is then compared to the score.

Instructions: This is a timed run to measure the heart and vascular system's capability to transport oxygen. It is an important area for performing police tasks involving stamina and endurance and to minimize the risk of cardiovascular problems. The score is in minutes and seconds.

Procedure: It is aerobic power test; the term "aerobics" was adopted from the term "aerobic" which refers to the type of metabolism utilizing oxygen in the production of energy for the body. The 12-minute run/walk test is used to determine the efficiency of the cardio-respiratory system.

Scoring: The total time taken for 12 minutes run/walk test was recorded as final score.

Important Suggestions Related to the Administration of the 12 Minutes Run/Walk Test:

i)   It was advised to maintain pace to avoid fatigue, practice running and pacing prior to the test.

ii)   Allow adequate time for stretching and warm-up exercises.

iii)   During the test, time will be called-out.

iv)   Guide them run according to their best of capability and endurance and do not over load yourself during course of the run. In case, continuous run is not possible, they may walk at their convenient distance and again they may resume running as per their convenience

v)   Do not disturb and talk to the other subjects so they may perform better and as per their level of capability.

vi)   It was instructed that one minute before a whistle will blow to indicate about the remaining time to motivate for the best coverage during one minute time.

vii)   At the finishing time, a long whistle will blow to indicate to stop as it is form and where is your position. It was also indicated that nobody should run or walk after the final whistle.

v)   Cool down; keep walking for five to ten minutes after the run to prevent pooling of blood in the lower extremities.

5. FLEXIBILITY- SIT AND REACH TEST

Purpose: To assess flexibility

Objective: To bend and reach as fast as possible. The standard flexibility tests that measures lower back and hamstring flexibility.

Equipment: It requires a box about 30cm (12 inches) high and a meter rule.

Instructions: **Sit and Reach Test:**

Procedure: Use these flexibility tests before you begin a stretching program and then every 6-8 weeks during your flexibility training. Before you perform these tests make sure you warm up thoroughly with 10 minutes of light jogging or skipping.

Scoring: The score is in the centimeters reached on a yardstick.

Important Suggestions Related to the Administration of the Sit and Reach Test:

1.Sit on the floor with your back and head against a wall. Legs should be out straight ahead and knees flat against the floor.

2.   Have someone place the box flat against your feet (no shoes). Keeping your back and head against the wall stretch your arms out towards the box.

3.   Have someone place the ruler on the box and move the zero ends towards your fingertips. When the ruler touches you fingertips you have the zero point and the test can begin.

4.   Lean forward slowly as far as possible keeping the fingertips level with each other and the legs flat. Your head and shoulders can come away from the wall now. Do not jerk or bounce to reach further.

5.   Slowly reach along the length of the ruler 3 times. On the third attempt reach as far as possible and hold for 2 seconds. Repeat twice and recorded the best score.

6. ONE MINUTE SIT-UPS TEST:

Purpose: To measure abdominal strength. This is a measure of the muscular endurance of the abdominal muscles. It is an important area for performing police tasks that may involve the use of force and is also an important area for maintaining good posture and minimizing lower back problems.

Equipment: Duties were spread on the ground and used for this purpose. Stop watch was used for noting time.

Procedure: The subject lay on his back with knees bend, feet on the floor, and heels not more than 12 inches from the buttocks. The subject puts his hand on the back of the neck with finger clasped and places elbows squarely on the mat. Feet were held by the partner to keep then in contact with surface. The subject tightened his abdominal muscle and brought head and elbow to the knees. This constituted one sit-up. He returned to the starting position with elbow on the surface before he started. On the command of 'GO' the subject started the sit-up. The performance was stopped on the word stop.

7. **Scoring:** The number of correct executed sit-ups performed in sixty seconds was the score or the score is in the number of bent leg sit-ups performed in one minute.

8. **PSYCHOMOTOR ABILITY- EYE HAND COORDINATION TEST:**

Purpose: To assess the eye-hand coordination of the subjects.

Objective: To complete the assigned task as fast as possible accurately.

Equipment: Psychomotor sheet (attached as appendix), pencil and Casio stop watch

Instructions: The subjects were asked to complete the line in between the two interlinked squares without lifting the pencil and touching the either line of the squares.

Procedure: The subjects were asked to sit comfortably on the desk or chair without any hurdles to write on the table. After the important instructions, first they were asked to complete the example given on the sheet, when they well understand the procedure How to do the task? Than they were asked to follow the command of the scholar/teacher, when they told to start the work and when asked to stop they have to stop at once and put the pencil and sheet separately. The total of five minutes was given to do the assigned work or complete the maximum possible squares correctly.

Scoring: The squares were tested with the help of magnifier, if any line of the square was touched or break in between the line that was not counted. Only correct squares were included in the final score.

9. CONCENTRATION- GRID CONCENTRATION TEST:

Purpose: To assess concentration ability.

Objective: To find-out the counting in sequence wise as fast as possible and cross with pencil.

Equipment: Grid test sheet for all the subjects, pencil, and Casio stop watch.

Instructions: Follow the instructions of the scholar, mind the command of start and stop, find the counting sequence wise and cross that with pencil.

Procedure: All the subjects were asked to follow the instructions, after giving the Grid test sheets asked   to find out the counting in sequence like 1, 2, 3, 4, 5, 6... and cross them with the help of pencil. The counting was written on the sheets from 1 to 100 in jumbled form.

Scoring: The sequence crossed counting was included in the final score. If left out any sequence one mark was reduced in the score.

10   SPORT COMPETITION ANXIETY TEST (SCAT)

Purpose:-

The sports Competition Anxiety Test is latest and most popular sport-specific anxiety test whose purpose is to assess individual differences in sports competitive trait anxiety or the tendency to pursue competition situations, as threatening, and /or to respond to these situations with elevated state anxiety.

Sports competition anxiety test questionnaire (SCAT) prepared by Rainer Martens (1986), was originally constructed for children (ages 10-15), its adult version was developed later on by suitably modifying the instructions and items. A reliability quotient of 0.85 had been reported for the adult version of SCAT.

Procedure:-

The SCAT questionnaire (Appendix-A) contains fifteen items. The subjects were asked to indicate how they generally felt in competitive sports situations, and responded to each item using a three point ordinal scale (hardly ever, sometimes, or often).

Out of fifteen items, only ten items assess sports competitive trait anxiety proneness (e.g., "Before I compete I feel uneasy") and used for scoring purpose. These ten items were: 2, 3, 5, 6, 8, 9, 11, 12, 14, and 15. The remaining five test items were the spurious items, which were added to the questionnaire to diminish response bias towards the actual test items (e.g., "Competing against others is socially enjoyable"). These five spurious items were not scored. These spurious were: 1, 4, 7, 10 and 13.

Every statement had three possible responses i.e.:-

1. Hardly ever
2. Sometimes
3. Often

69

While the subjects were responding to the questionnaire, the scholar went around verifying that they were recording answers sequentially and explained the meaning of the words in case of doubts.

Scoring:-

The scholar scrutinized the completed questionnaire in order to ensure that the subject responds to every item and there was no question left unanswered. The items 2, 3, 5, 8, 9, 12, 14 and 15 were worded in such a manner that they were scored according to the following key:-

ScoreResponse	
1	Hardly ever
2	Sometimes
3	Often

In the case of items 6 and 11 scoring was carried out according to the following key:-

Score	Response
1	Often
2	Sometime
3	Hardly ever

However spurious questions i.e. 1, 4, 7, 10, and 13 were not be scored as suggested by Rainer Martens.

If a subject deleted one of the test items, her prorated full scale score was obtained by computing the mean score for the nine items answered, multiplying this value by ten values by ten, and rounding the product to the next whole number. When two or more items were omitted, the respondent's questionnaire was invalidated.

Total scores of SCAT ranged from 10 (low competitive anxiety) to 30 (high competitive anxiety). The subjects were assigned to the following category according to the score obtained by them:

Raw/Mean Score	Classification
Less than 17	Low Anxieties
17 – 24	Moderate Anxiety
More than 24	High Anxiety

Responses obtained from the subjects on each statements of sports competition anxiety questionnaires were subjected to statistical treatment keeping in view the purpose of study.

Sport-Confidence Inventory
Purpose:-

To measure sport self-confidence Sports Self Confidence Inventory (Appendix -B) prepared by Robin S. Vealy (1986) was used for this study Questions were based on how confident players generally felt when they competed in sports. They compared their self-confidence to the most confident athlete the knew. A reliability quotient of 0.73 was reported for the Sport Confidence Inventory.

Procedure:-

Sport confidence inventory has thirteen items. There are no rights or wrong answers in the inventory. Every question has nine possible responses, i.e. 1 to 3 low, 4 to 6 medium, 7 to 9 high. The subjects were instructed to respond to each question how they felt by placing a circle on the appropriate response.

Scoring:-

The scholar scrutinized the completed questionnaires in order to ensure that that the subjects respond to every item and there was no question left unanswered. The level of self-confidence depends upon the score obtained. The subjects were assigned to the following categories according to the scores obtained by them:

Raw/Mean Score	Classification
13 – 47	Low Self –Confidence
48 – 82	Moderate Self-Confidence
83 – 117	High Self-Confidence

Responses obtained from the subjects on each statement of self confidence inventory were recorded for analysis of data.

TABLE - 2

TESTER'S RELIABILITY THROUGH COEFFICIENTS OF CORRELATION

S. No.	Variables / Test Items	'r' Value
1	Body Mass Index	0.88
2	40 m Dash (in Secs.)	0.97
3	Standing Broad Jump (in cms.)	0.95
4	Sit & Reach Test (in cms.)	0.90
5	Sit-ups Test (in count)	0.98
6	12 Min. Run/Walk Test (in m.)	0.92
7	Psycho-motor Ability Test	0.89
8	Grid Test	0.95
9.	SCAT-Test	0.96

Instrumental Reliability:

For the purpose of the test all the instruments were used of high standard and reputed companies and were calibrated by the respective companies. The stop watches were used from Casio Company make.

All the instruments were calibrated prior to the actual testing procedure with the help of experts and also gone through the several practice trials with instruments and testing.

Therefore, it was well established reliability of the instruments used in the present study.

Statistical Procedure:

For the purpose of the analyses, the following statistical procedures were employed:

In first step, descriptive statistics was employed in which Mean; SD, Minimum and Maximum scores were computed. The required statistical calculations were computed with the help of SPSS software. The descriptive calculation and 't' test were computed. Then, both the groups were tested to observe the differences among the selected variables.

The level of significance was set at .05 level of confidence.

CHAPTER - IV

ANALYSIS OF DATA AND RESULTS
OF THE STUDY

Introduction:

The present study was designed to assess the psycho-motor abilities of Kabaddi and Kho-Kho players of Delhi Schools. The psycho-motor abilities were identified and selected with the specific variables and their relevant test items. The selected tests were administered as per the testing protocol and scores were recorded as a raw data. The raw data were statistically analysed to find-out the results of the study, which has been presented in this chapter.

The data of selected tests items related to motor ability and psychological aspects have been taken such as: Body Mass Index showing level of physical fitness, 40 m Dash for Speed, Standing Broad Jump for Explosive Strength, One minutes Sit-ups for Muscular Strength, Sit and Reach Test for Trunk and Legs Flexibility, 12 Minutes Run/Walk for Endurance, Psycho-motor Test for Eye-hand Coordination, Grid Test for Concentration and Sports Competition Anxiety Test (SCAT) to assess the level of anxiety of Kabaddi and Kho-Kho players were collected on one hundred male players, who were first three position holder at Zonal, Inter Zonal, and participated in the National Schools games (SGFI) or participated in Junior National Championship in year 2009-2010.

The present study was conducted to observe and find-out the differences among all the selected motor ability and psychological variables. The data were collected in raw form and analyzed by computing the descriptive statistical techniques and 't' test were applied. The level of significance was set at .05 level of confidence.

Results of the Study:

The differences among Kabaddi and Kho-Kho players of Delhi schools were observed on selected physical and psychological variables. The required statistical calculations were computed with the help of SP&SS software. The calculations of descriptive statistics and 't' test results had been computed and tabulated in accordance with the selected variables. Each variable was taken-up with the help of data and requisite table. Further, each table was also analyzed to project the results in view of the objectives, delimitations and hypothesis etc. The table, analysis and graphical representations were presented to project and for better understanding. These were presented in Table: 3 to Table: 7. The graphical presentations of the mean values of mean of selected nine variables in Figure: 1 to Figure: 9

TABLE: 3
DESCRIPTIVE STATISTICS OF SELECTED VARIABLES FOR KABADDI AND KHO-KHO PLAYERS

S. NO.	VARIABLES	MEAN-KABADDI	MEAN-KHO-KHO	MEAN DIFFERENCE
1	Body Mass Index	22.09	19.65	02.44
2	40 M Dash (in secs.)	7.62	6.61	01.01
3	Standing Broad Jump (in cms.)	2.08	1.89	0.19
4	Sit & Reach Test (in cms.)	16.58	21.40	04.82
5	Sit-ups Test (in count)	38.10	32.68	05.42
6	12 min. Run/Walk Test (inmts.)	1691.5	2088.8	397.3
7	Psychomotor Ability Test	34.04	38.12	04.08
8	Grid Test	14.94	16.24	01.3
9.	SCAT Test	14.12	16.78	02.66

N =100 (50 Kabaddi & 50 Kho-Kho)

The Table - 3 highlight the mean values of Kabaddi and Kho-Kho players for the selected variables. The Body Mass Index for Kabaddi players depicts 22.09 and Kho-Kho players 19.65 with a mean difference of 02.44. It shows that Kabaddi players have more BMI score or they were fatter than the Kho-Kho players. The mean value for 40 M Dash for Kabaddi and Kho-Kho players were 7.62 and 6.61 seconds respectively with a difference of 1.01 seconds, signifying that Kho-Kho players were reported faster than the Kabaddi players.

FIGURE: 1

GRAPHICAL PRESENTATION OF COMPARATIVE MEAN VALUE
OF BODY MASS INDEX OF KABADDI AND KHO-KHO PLAYERS

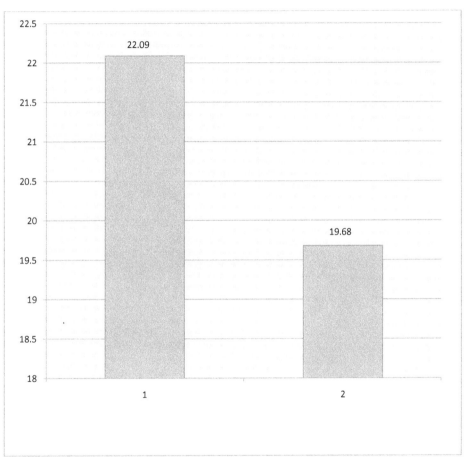

The Figure: 4.01 indicate the projection of comparative mean values Kabaddi (1) and Kho-Kho (2) players in reference to Body Mass Index. It is clearly evident that Kabaddi players have more BMI than the Kho-Kho players

FIGURE: 2
GRAPHICAL PRESENTATION OF COMPARATIVE MEAN VALUES OF 40 M DASH FOR KABADDI AND KHO-KHO PLAYERS (IN SECONDS)

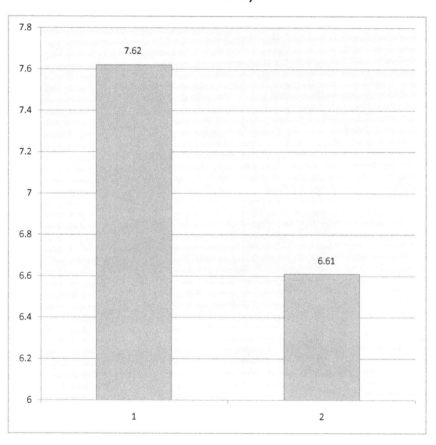

The Figure: 2 represent the comparative Mean Values of 40 M Dash Test Item for Kabaddi and Kho-Kho players. The lesser timings means better performancehence, Kho-Kho (2) players have better sprinting ability than the Kabaddi (1) players.

FIGURE: 3

GRAPHICAL PRESENTATION OF COMPARATIVE MEAN VALUES OF STANDING BROAD JUMP OF KABADDI AND KHO-KHO PLAYERS

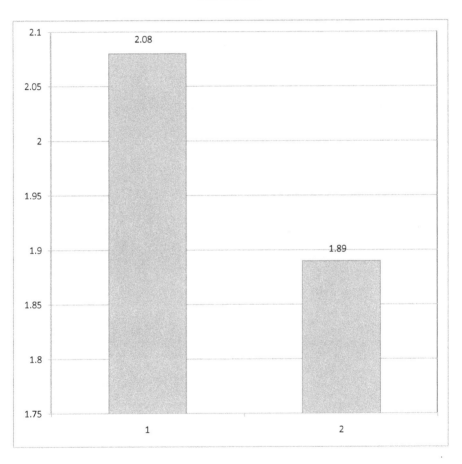

The Figure: 3 exhibits the comparative mean values for Standing Broad Jump as 2.08 M and 1.89 M respectively with a difference of 0.19 M. It clearly indicates from the data and said figure that Kabaddi players have more Explosive Leg Strength than Kho-Kho players.

FIGURE: 4

GRAPHICAL PRESENTATION OF COMPARATIVE MEAN VALUE OFSIT AND REACH TEST OF KABADDI AND KHO-KHO PLAYERS

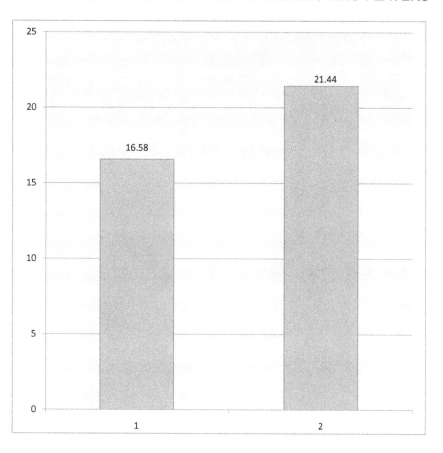

Figure: 4 highlight the status of comparative mean values for Kabaddi and Kho-Kho players for the Sit and Reach Test Item as: 16.58 and 21.40 respectively with amean difference of 4.82. It clearly shows that the Kho-Kho players have better flexibility than Kabaddi players.

FIGURE: 5

GRAPHICAL PRESENTATION OF COMPARATIVE MEAN VALUES OF SIT-UPS OF KABADDI AND KHO-KHO PLAYERS

Figure: 5 represent the comparative mean value status of One Minutes Sit-ups Test for Kabaddi and Kho-Kho players which were measured in count as: 38.10 and 32.68 respectively with a mean difference of 5.42. It indicates that Kabaddi playershave more strength endurance for abdominal muscles.

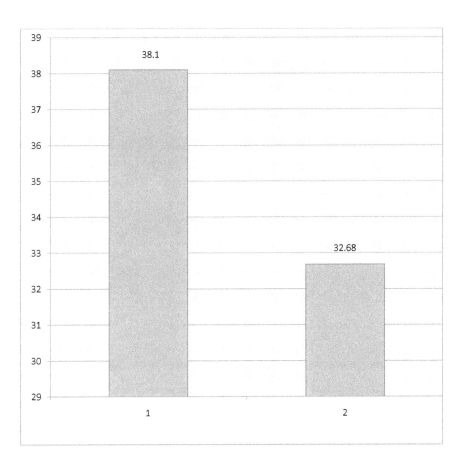

Figure: 6

GRAPHICAL PRESENTATION OF COMPARATIVE MEAN VALUES OF 12 MINUTES RUN/WALK OF KABADDI AND KHO-KHO PLAYERS

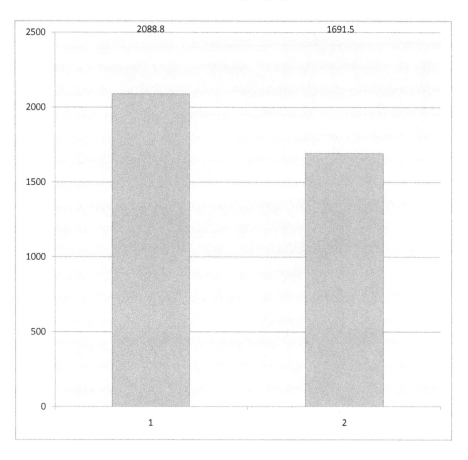

Figure: 6 The general cardiovascular endurance was tested with a standardized test of 12min Run/Walk test, which measured mean value 1691.5 meters and 2088.8 meters with difference of 397.3 meters in favor of Kho-Kho players, mean the Kho-Kho players had better cardiovascular endurance.

FIGURE: 7

GRAPHICAL PRESENTATION OF COMPARATIVE MEAN VALUES OF PSYCHO-MOTOR ABILITY OF KABADDI AND KHO-KHO PLAYERS

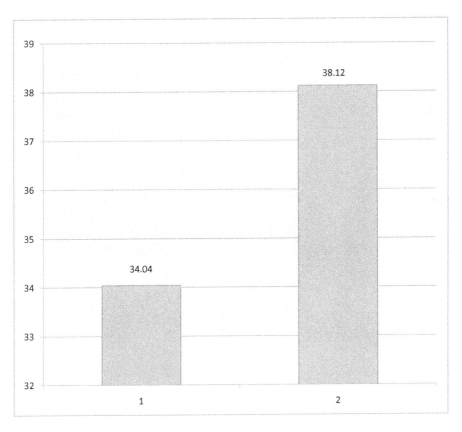

Figure: 7 represents the graphical representation of comparative mean values related to psycho-motor ability recorded through data of Kabaddi and Kho-Kho players of Delhi Schools. The means computed as: 34.04 and 38.12 for Kabaddi and Kho-Kho players respectively with a difference of 4.08. It may be observed that Kho-Kho players were better in Eye-hand Coordination Ability.

FIGURE: 8

GRAPHICAL PRESENTATION OF COMPARATIVE MEAN VALUES OF CONCENTRATION ABILITYOF KABADDI AND KHO-KHO PLAYERS

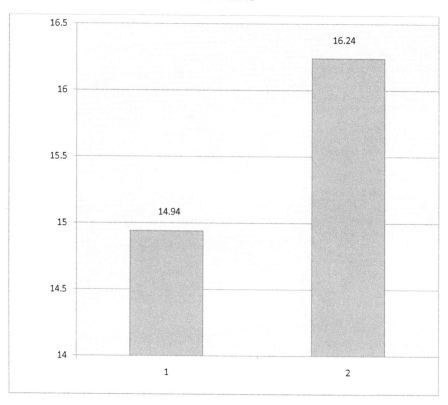

Figure: 8 indicate the status of comparative mean values of Mental Concentration Ability for Kabaddi and Kho-Kho players of Delhi Schools which was measured through Grid Test for Concentration. The mean scores for Kabaddi players were 14.94 and for Kho-Kho were 16.24 with a mean difference of 1.3. It may be observed that Kho-Kho players had better scores in Concentration means they require more concentration than the Kabaddi players.

FIGURE: 9

GRAPHICAL PRESENTATION OF COMPARATIVE MEAN VALUES OF SPORTS COMPETITION ANXIETY LEVEL FOR KABADDI AND KHO-KHO PLAYERS

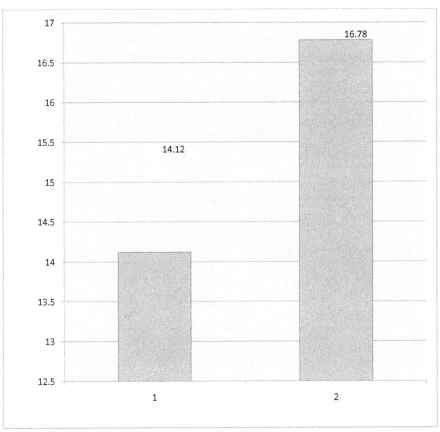

Figure: 9 represents the comparative mean scores of Kabaddi and Kho-Kho players for Sports Competition Anxiety Test (SCAT, Marten, 1977) was administered and found that mean values for Kabaddi was 14.12 and for Kho-Kho was 16.78 with a difference of 2.66. On the basis of scores, it may be stated that the level of anxiety was found more in Kho-Kho players.

TABLE: 4
DESCRIPTIVE STATISTICS OF KABADDI PLAYERS OF
SELECTED VARIABLES

S. NO.	VARIABLES	MINIMUM SCORES	MAXIMUM SCORES
1	Body Mass Index	18.4	24.8
2	40 M Dash (in sec.)	6.45	9.89
3	Standing Broad Jump (in cm)	1.48	2.53
4	Sit & Reach Test (in cm)	09	26
5	Sit-ups Test (in count)	17	52
6	12 Min. Run Test (in mts.)	1145	2340
7	Psycho-motor Test	19	46
8	Grid Test	08	23
9.	SCAT Test	08	18

N =50

Table: 4.02 highlights the comparative scores (Minimum and Maximum) of Kabaddi players for each test item selected for the present study. The minimum and maximum scores of Kabaddi players were for BMI 18.4 & 24.8, 40 M Dash 6.45 sec. & 9.89 sec., Standing Broad Jump 1.48 m & 2.53 m, Sit and Reach 09 cm & 26 cm, Sit-ups 17 & 52, 12 Min. Run/Walk Test with a distance of 1145 m & 2340 m, Psycho-motor Test for Eye-hand Coordination 19 & 23, Grid Test for Concentration 08 & 23 and SCAT for Sports Competition Anxiety 08 & 18.

TABLE: 5
DESCRIPTIVE STATISTICS OF KHO-KHO PLAYERS OF SELECTED VARIABLES

S. NO.	VARIABLES	MINIMUM SCORES	MAXIMUM SCORES
1	Body Mass Index	17.4	22.4
2	40 M Dash (in sec.)	5.46	8.65
3	Standing Broad Jump (in cm)	1.32	2.39
4	Sit & Reach Test (in cm)	13	37
5	Sit-ups Test (in count)	15	43
6	12 Min. Run Test (in mts.)	1270	2625
7	Psycho-motor Test	22	50
8	Grid Test	9	24
9	SCAT Test	12	24

N =50

The Table: 4.03 exhibit the minimum and maximum scores of Kho-Kho players for selected variables were reported like: BMI: 17.4 & 22.4, 40 M Dash: 5.46 sec. & 8.65 sec., Standing Broad Jump: 1.32 m & 2.39 m, Sit and Reach 13 cm & 37 cm, Sit-ups 15 & 43, 12 Min. Run/Walk Test Distance was 1270 M & 2625 M, Psycho-motor Test for Eye-hand Coordination 22 & 50, Grid Test for Concentration 09 & 24 and SCAT Test for Sports Competition Anxiety 12 & 24.

TABLE: 6

SIGNIFICANCE OF MEAN COMPARISON OF SELECTED VARIABLES

S. No.	Variables	Paired Mean Difference	Paired S. D. Difference	't' Value
1	Body Mass Index	2.45	2.43	7.11**
2	40m Dash	1.01	1.21	5.89**
3	Standing Broad Jump	.19	.311	4.24**
4	Sit & Reach Test	4.86	6.94	4.96**
5	Sit-ups Test	5.42	7.25	5.29**
6	12min. Run Test	3.98	500.75	5.61**
7	Psychomotor Test	4.08	6.24	4.62**
8	Grid Test	1.30	5.19	1.77
9.	SCAT-Test	2.66	4.14	4.54**

*Significance at 0.05 level (df = 49) 2.01

**Significance at 0.01 level (df = 49) 2.68

The Table: 4.04 reflect the status of two tailed equal group statistical significance mean comparison for which 't' test was employed on both the sets of data Kabaddi and Kho-Kho players on selected variables with the help of SPSS, a computerized software meant for the statistical calculations for the data of social sciences including education and physical education.

The results mentioned in the Table: 4.04 in which it was found that for the Body Mass Index, the paired mean differences were 2.45, paired S.D. difference was 2.43 and 't' value was 7.11,which was highly significant at both 0.05 and 0.01 levels of confidence as the tabulated values depicted as 2.01 and 2.68 respectively. It may be observed from the results that there is a significant difference between Kabaddi and Kho-Kho players in reference to Body Mass Index component.

A test for measuring speed was selected as 40 M Dash for which the values of paired mean difference were 1.01, paired S.D. difference was 1.21 and 't' value was 5.89 was significant at both 0.05 and 0.01 levels of confidence against the tabulated value 2.01 and 2.68 respectively. It may also be observed that the speed component has significant difference between Kabaddi and Kho-Kho Players.

The paired mean difference for Standing Broad Jump was 0.19, paired S.D. difference was 0.31 and 't' value was 4.24,which was found significant at both 0.05 and 0.01 levels of confidence. The Sit & Reach Test was computed for the paired mean difference which were 4.86, paired S.D. difference 6.94 and 't' value was 4.96 was significant at both 0.05 and 0.01 levels of confidence against the tabulated value 2.01 and 2.68 respectively.

The Table: 4.04 also indicates about the test of one minutes Sit-ups with the paired mean difference was reported as: 5.42, paired S.D. difference was computed

7.25 and 't' value was 5.29, was found significant at both 0.05 and 0.01 levels of confidence. The cardio-vascular endurance was tested through 12 minute Run/Walk Test. The paired mean difference was 3.98, paired S.D. difference was computed 500.75 and 't' value was calculatedas 5.61,which was reported as significant at both 0.05 and 0.01 levels of confidence against the tabulated values: 2.01 and 2.68 respectively.

The Psycho-motor ability was reported that the paired mean difference were 4.08, paired S.D. difference 6.24 and 't' value was 4.62,which may be observed as significant at both 0.05 and 0.01 levels of confidence against the tabulated value of 2.01 and 2.68 respectively.

For testing the mental concentration, a Grid Test was applied and found that the paired mean difference were 1.30, paired S.D. difference 5.19 and 't' value was 1.77, which was not found significant at either levels of confidence. Because its calculated 't' value was lesser than the tabulated value i.e. 2.01. It clearly indicates that there is no significant difference between the Kabaddi and Kho-Kho players in reference to mental concentration which means that in both the sports players must have the close level of mental concentration.

The Sports Competition Anxiety Test (SCAT) was administered and it was found that the paired mean difference were 2.66, paired S.D. difference 4.14 and 't' value was 4.54,which was found significant at both 0.05 and 0.01 levels of confidence against the tabulated values of 2.01 and 2.68 respectively.

Discussion on the Findings

To find-out the psycho-motor differences between Kabaddi and Kho-Kho players of Delhi Schools on their selected Physical and Psychological variables. The required statistical calculations were computed with the help of SPSS software. The difference among all the selected motor abilities and psychological variables, the data were collected and analyzed by using the descriptive statistics and 't' test as statistical techniques. The level of significance was set at .05. When, a two tailed equal group statistical significance mean comparison 't' test was employed on both the sets of data related to the Kabaddi and Kho-Kho players on selected variables.

The 't' value for Body Mass Index was 7.11,which was found significant at both 0.05 and 0.01 levels of confidence. It was signifying that the Kabaddi players were found heavier and fatty, which is also required for better Kabaddi performance. A Kabaddi player needs to stop, pull, push and drag the opponents with his strength and muscular weight. Therefore, they required to put optimum bodyweight/fat (maximum body weight permitted as 80kg.) for their best possible performance in contrary to the Kho-Kho players.

The speed test was conducted as 40 M Dash and the 't' value was 5.89, which was also found significant at both 0.05 and 0.01 levels of confidence against the tabulated values of 2.01 and 2.68 respectively, while the degree of freedom was 1/49. It showed and proved that the Kho-Kho players were faster than Kabaddi players. As Kho-Kho players need to dash or all out sprint for 15-20 meters frequently in their practice and competition. Therefore, their acceleration speed is better than the Kabaddi players, which a basic requirement to be Kho-Kho competitive player.

The 't' value of Standing Broad Jump was 4.24,which was found significant at both 0.05 and 0.01 levels with the mean difference of 0.19 which showed that Kabaddi players have more explosive leg strength than Kho-Kho players. As, explosive strength ability is widely accepted motor ability of Kabaddi players, they have to jump in almost all directions to save themselves from the opponents and out them. Sometimes, they have to jump over the opponents, back jump to touch the center line, side sift to self-save etc. It may be observed that Kabaddi players have significant difference with Kho-Kho players, which means Kabaddi players have better explosive strength ability.

The Sit & Reach test was considered to assess the flexibility of the Kabaddi and Kho-Kho players of Delhi schools. The 't' ratio was computed and found the value as 4.96,which seems significant at both 0.05 and 0.01 levels of confidence. The mean values were 16.58 cm and 21.40 cm for Kabaddi and Kho-Kho players respectively with a mean difference of 4.82 cm sign of better flexibility in Kho-Kho players. It may be due to Kabaddi players emphasize less on flexibility exercises or Kho-Kho players need to move in different direction quickly, sit and run to chase opponents. Therefore, they have to perform more flexibility exercises in practice sessions to give their best possible performance in competition.

The one minute Sit-ups test was conducted to assess the strength endurance of abdominal muscles. The difference was sought among Kabaddi and Kho-Kho players with the help of 't' ratio which was calculated with a value of 5.29.It was found significant at both 0.05 and 0.01 levels of confidence. The one minute Sit-ups test was measured in count with a mean value for the players of Kabaddi 38.10 and Kho-Kho 32.68 with the mean difference of 5.42 which shows that Kabaddi players had more strength endurance for abdominal muscles. They put more efforts to develop the strength endurance, which is an ultimate requirement too for the Kabaddi players.

The Cardio-vascular Endurance was measured through 12 Minute Run/Walk Test conducted on Kabaddi and Kho-Kho players of Delhi schools. To assess the difference in composite performance of Kabaddi and Kho-Kho players, the 't' ratio was computed which was calculated with a value of 5.61.The significant values were set at both 0.05 and 0.01 levels of confidence against the tabulated value which depicted as 2.01 and 2.68 respectively.

To evaluate the cardio-vascular endurance, a test of 12min Run/Walk was conducted. The composite scores of the test were measured with mean values as 1691.5 meters and 2088.8 meters with a difference of 397.3 meters. The comparative mean value was found in favor of Kho-Kho players. The mean more for the Kho-Kho players signifying they had better cardiovascular endurance than Kho-Kho players. It is because, the Kho-Kho players had to run and escaped from the chaser for maximum of 9 minutes with high intensity. So, they have to put more efforts to develop and maintained the endurance for their best possible performance in competition.

The Psycho-motor ability was assessed to find-out the difference on the composite performances of Kabaddi and Kho-Kho players. The 't' value was computed 4.62, which was again found significant at both 0.05 and 0.01 levels of confidence against tabulated values were 2.01 and 2.68 respectively. A test of psycho-motor ability was tested with mean values 34.04 and 38.12 for Kabaddi and Kho-Kho players respectively with a difference of 4.08 which clearly evident that Kho-Kho players were better in eye-hand coordination. They had better abilities of steadiness and mental-physical coordination than Kabaddi players due to emphasized on these types of exercises.

For mental concentration a test namely- Grid Test was applied and found the 't' value 1.77, which was not found significant at 0.05 level of confidence. Because its calculated 't' value was less than the tabulated value 2.01. It may be due to the similar type of concentration ability among the Kabaddi and Kho-Kho players. The mental concentration ability was measured with grid test of concentration with mean for Kabaddi 14.94 and Kho-Kho 16.24 with mean difference of 1.84 showed that Kho-Kho players had better scores in concentration, but there was no significant difference.

The Sports Competition Anxiety Test (SCAT) on administered ON Kabaddi and Kho-Kho players. To assess the difference with the help of 't' ratio, the value was computed as 4.54,which was found to be significant at both 0.05 and 0.01 levels of confidence as the tabulated values were 2.01 and 2.68 respectively. The mean value found for Kabaddi 14.12 and Kho-Kho 16.78 with a difference of 2.66 showed Kho-Kho players had more anxiety. An optimum level of stress and anxiety is necessary for optimum / best possible level sports performance. It was found that both the games players found normal level of anxiety but Kho-Kho players little high level of anxiety than the Kabaddi players may be due to situational aspect and mood state of the players at the time of administration of the test as per the limitation of the study.

CHAPTER- V
SUMMARY, CONCLUSIONS AND RECOMMENDATIONS

Summary

The main objective of the present study was to compare the Kabaddi and Kho-Kho players of Delhi schools, who has obtained position at Zonal and Inter-zonal and participated in National School Games' (SGFI) respective sports competition on selected physical and psychological abilities through the selected test items such as: Body Mass Index (BMI), Speed, Standing Broad Jump, Sit and Reach, Sit-ups, 12 Minutes Run/walk, Psycho-motor Ability Test, Concentration Ability and Sports Competition Anxiety Test between the players of Kabaddi and Kho-Kho.

For the purpose of the present study, finally one hundred players were selected as subjects. Out of total one hundred subjects, 50 subjects from the game of Kabaddi and 50 subjects from the Kho-Kho has been selected on purposive and random sampling basis, who has won medal/position in Delhi schools' tournaments like: zonal, Inter-zonal and participated in National School Games (SGFI) during the 2009 and 2010. All the subjects were involved in regular practice as a preparation for their targeted competition in their respective sports. The selected subjects were voluntarily agreed to become as the subjects and promised to cooperate during the course of the study and collection of data.

The research scholar gleaned through all the scientific literature pertaining to Kabaddi and Kho-Kho from books, magazines, journals, periodicals available at various libraries of Delhi and internet websites. The scholar visited numerous libraries where there was a possibility to locate the related literature. The scholar visited the libraries like: Indira Gandhi Institute of Physical Education & Sports Sciences: University of Delhi, Central Library: University of Delhi, Central Institute of Education: University of Delhi, National Council for Educational Research and Training: New Delhi, Laxmibal National University of Physical Education: Gwalior (MP) etc. to search the relevant literature and reviews for the present study. Keeping in view, the feasibility criterion in mind, especially in the case of availability of instruments, the test items for testing the following psycho-physical abilities were considered and selected i.e. Body Mass Index (BMI), Speed, Standing Broad Jump, Sit and Reach, Sit-ups, 12 Minutes Run/Walk, Psycho-motor Ability, Concentration ability and Sports Competition Anxiety Test.

The testing protocol of each selected test item was followed carefully for administration of test in a correct and required manner. The reliability of testers and instruments were also established before the start of the data collection. The necessary data was collected with standardized procedure by administering selected psychophysical ability tests as suggested by Hardyal Singh and W. Cooper etc.

The necessary work was done before the start of the test. Firstly, the practice sessions were administered several times of each test with the help of the Supervisor, experts and required support staff etc. All the tests were administered and explained to the subjects by the scholar categorically and left no ambiguity. In case of any doubt raised by the subjects were clarified before taking the test, but no special training was given to the subjects.

The tests were administered and data were recorded as the raw data. To find-out the difference between Kabaddi and Kho-Kho players of Delhi schools on their selected Physical and Psychological variables, the required statistical calculations were computed with the help of SPSS software. The difference among all the selected motor abilities and psychological variables, the data were collected and analysed by using the descriptive statistics and 't' test. The level of significance was set at .05. When a two tailed equal group statistical significance mean comparison 't' test was employed on both the set of data Kabaddi and Kho-Kho players on selected variables, the results evident significant in majority of the variables.

The following variables were found significant at both 0.05 and 0.01 level of confidence such as: Body Mass Index: 't' value 7.11,Speed Test by 40 M Dash: 't' value 5.89,Standing Broad Jump: the 't' value 4.24, Sit & Reach test: 't' value 4.96,the test of strength endurance- One minute Sit-ups: the 't' value 5.29, Cardio-vascular Endurance in the form of 12 Minutes Run/Walk Test, the 't' value was 5.61,which were significant at both 0.05 and 0.01 level.

The Psychomotor Ability computed the 't' value as 4.62andSports Competition Anxiety Test (SCAT) was found with 't' value as 4.54, which was significant at both 0.05 and 0.01 level of confidence, while the tabulated value 2.01 and 2.68 respectively.

Whereas, the Mental Concentration Ability was tested through a test namely: Grid Test was applied and found with the 't' value 1.77, which was not found significant difference at 0.05 level of confidence. Because its calculated 't' value was less than the tabulated value. It may be due to the similar type of Concentration Ability among the Kabaddi and Kho-Kho players.

The Mental Concentration Ability was measured through Grid Test for concentration showed that Kho-Kho players had better scores than the Kabaddi players in mental concentration ability, but there was no significant difference found. It was observed that the level of mental concentration have a close requirement for the Kabaddi and Kho-Kho players.

The Kho-Kho players had reported higher level of anxiety than Kabaddi players. An optimum level of stress and anxiety were observed which indicate about the necessity for optimum / best possible level of sports performance. It was also observed that both Kabaddi and Kho-Kho players found normal level of anxiety. But, Kho-Kho players had little higher level of anxiety than the Kabaddi players which may be due to situational aspect and mood state of the players at the time of administration of the test. Further, the said situation may be considered as one of the limitation of the study.

The data were presented in requisite tables as per the requirement of the delimitations, objectives and selection of the variables. The tables were presented along with the relevant analysis which were also supported the graphical representations. The scholar has drawn certain conclusions out of the findings of the present study and suggested some recommendations for the future research, which may be conducted in related area.

Conclusions:

On the basis of the data analysis, limitations and findings of the present study, the following conclusions were drawn:

1. The significant difference was found in the Body Mass Index- in relation to the Kabaddi and Kho-Kho players. The Kabaddi players' group was found with a higher level of BMI which shows greater body mass than the Kho-Kho players' group.

2. The significant difference was found in the Speed Ability tested through 40 M Dash Test. The Kho-Kho players' group had better speed in comparison to the Kabaddi players' group.

3. The significant difference was found in the Standing Broad Jump, a test of explosive strength in relation to the Kabaddi and Kho-Kho players. The Kabaddi players' group had better explosive strength, showing greater jumping ability than the Kho-Kho players' group.

4. The significant difference was found in the Sit and Reach Test. The Kho-Kho players' group had better hips and legs flexibility in comparison to the Kabaddi players' group.

5. The significant difference was found in the One Minute Sit-ups, a test to measure muscular strength endurance in relation to the Kabaddi and Kho-Kho players. The Kabaddi players' group had better muscular strength endurance of abdomen muscles group, showing greater muscular endurance ability than the Kho-Kho players' group.

6. The significant difference was found in the 12 Minutes Run/Walk Test of Cardio-vascular Endurance in relation to the Kabaddi and Kho-Kho players. The Kho-Kho players' group had better Cardio-vascular Endurance, showing greater heart and lungs' capacity than the group of Kabaddi players.

7. The significant difference was found in the Psycho-motor Ability in relation to the Kabaddi and Kho-Kho players. The Kho-Kho players' group had better Psycho-motor Ability or Eye-hand Co-ordination, proving better mental and physical Coordinative Ability than the Kabaddi players.

8. There was no significant difference found in relation to Concentration Ability measured through Grid Test between Kabaddi and Kho-Kho players.

9. The significant difference was found in the Sports Competition Anxiety Test (SCAT) in relation to the Kabaddi and Kho-Kho players. The Kho-Kho players' group had higher level of anxiety than the selected group of Kabaddi players. Whereas, both the groups had optimum level of anxiety to perform better in their respective sports competitions.

Recommendations:

In light of the findings and conclusions drawn from the present study, the following recommendations were made for further academic and research pursuit in the field of physical education and sports:

1. The similar nature of studies may be undertaken on female players or counter part of male Kabaddi and Kho-Kho players.

2. The similar studies may be conducted by taking others variables which may affects the performance of the Kabaddi and Kho-Kho players along with others important variables such as: physical, physiological and psychological.

3. The similar nature of studies may also be undertaken by comparing the players of the other team games sports' competition.

4. Similar studies may be undertaken by comparing the players of the other team games sports' competition.

5. The similar nature of studies may also be undertaken by comparing the players of the individual sports' competition.

6. Similar studies may be undertaken by comparing the players belonging to different socio-economic status, geographical conditions and variation in ethnicity.

7. The same type of study can be conducted on other levels of players as subjects like: Senior National or International level.

8. It is also recommended that the training programme for Kabaddi and Kho-Kho players should be different as per their respective needs and requirements of the games.

9. The training for the speed and flexibility should not be neglected for the Kabaddi players as these are important factors to apply difficult technique in Kabaddi as well as to avoid injuries.

10. The safety precautions should always be adopted for the Kabaddi and Kho-Kho training and competition for the safety of the players.

11. A study may be undertaken with fully residential subjects of different age groups junior / senior, men and women, who should be regular in their preparation for the competitions.

CPSIA information can be obtained
at www.ICGtesting.com
Printed in the USA
BVHW050317200223
658797BV00011B/1939